MEDICARE TOMORROW

Medicare Tomorrow

The Report of
The Century Foundation
Task Force on Medicare Reform

With background papers by
Lisa Potetz and Thomas Rice

The Century Foundation Press • New York

The Century Foundation sponsors and supervises timely analyses of economic policy, foreign affairs, and domestic political issues. Not-for-profit and nonpartisan, it was founded in 1919 and endowed by Edward A. Filene.

LIBRARY OF CONGRESS CATALOGING-IN-PUBLICATION DATA
Medicare tomorrow : the report of the Century Foundation Task Force on Medicare Reform.
    p. cm.
  Includes bibliographical references and index.
  ISBN 0-87078-463-3 (pbk. : alk. paper)
  1. Medicare. 2. Health care reform—United States.   I. Century Foundation Task Force on Medicare Reform.
  RA412.3 .M446 2001
  368.2'26'00973—dc21

                                                2001004682

Manufactured in the United States of America.

FOREWORD

The United States is the wealthiest nation in the world and easily the biggest spender on medical care. Yet it is, by many measures, far from the healthiest nation. Without joining the debate about how to assess comparisons between the health of Americans and citizens of other developed nations, it is fair to say that many who deal with this complex area are uneasy, in some cases even alarmed, about the quality and cost of health care in the United States. Sorting through the reasons for these apparent deficiencies in health care is complicated. It helps to start by recognizing that there is, in fact, no single American health system. Instead, as in so many other areas, the United States has developed a complex system all its own, a special blend of public and private, national and local, excellent and mediocre.

One of the major flashpoints in the current debates about health care is the state of the nation's largest publicly supported health insurance program, Medicare. One basic point about the Medicare debate is quite straightforward: although there are those who would like to scrap the program completely and shift to a market-based system, people who actually run for office overwhelmingly talk about saving, not replacing, the program. Medicare, in other words, has strong political backing among the millions of Americans who depend upon it for health care.

There have been many reports in recent years about how to deal with various issues affecting Medicare. Nearly all, however, have focused on the financial aspects of the program. In fact, for more than a decade, because of the unprecedented peacetime deficits generated during the Reagan-Bush presidencies, virtually all national policy debates have been focused on budgetary and financial issues. Medicare, a large and rapidly growing federal "cost center," is no exception. And indeed, the problem of long-term federal budgeting was the centerpiece of the approach taken by the leadership of the President's National Bipartisan Commission on the Future of Medicare during 1998 and 1999.

This task force report shifts the focus away from financial issues—although they are undeniably important—toward the goals of the program. It emphasizes that Medicare has helped bring about increased economic security and better health for older and disabled Americans. It discusses how these goals may be best preserved and extended in the future. In this respect, the members' call for a prescription drug benefit within Medicare is especially timely, reaffirming as it does the importance of a collective social insurance framework for the Medicare program.

This approach also is critical because an increasing number of Americans will enter the program over the next few decades at the same time that beneficial but expensive medical therapies are certain to be developed. The members of the task force agreed that Medicare's commitments are worth preserving despite the higher price tag that the program almost certainly will carry in the future, and they placed this spending in the appropriate context of Medicare's importance to seniors, the disabled, and their families. The report makes it clear that Medicare spending is inescapably about our basic social values, and it lays out a series of principles that offer guidelines for in-depth evaluations of the reform proposals that have been suggested.

The Century Foundation has been concerned with issues of health care and health insurance coverage since its inception. It sponsored research that helped lay the groundwork for the evolution of group health insurance in the United States. More recently, we have published a guide to the issues involved in the debate in our series, the Basics—*Medicare Reform*—and we have supported publication of an edited volume on aging in the United States, *Life in an Older America;* a study by Charles Morris, *Too Much of a Good Thing?* on how health care spending is valued; and a book by Joseph White, *False Alarm,* that challenges the conventional wisdom that Social Security and Medicare are in a precarious financial condition. Our ongoing work in this area includes an examination of these issues by Henry Aaron and Robert Reischauer.

The members of the Task Force on Medicare Reform, which was chaired by Shoshanna Sofaer and Richard Ravitch, gave freely of their time and knowledge. While perhaps no member agrees with every line in the report that follows, the document does represent an important consensus among a diverse and distinguished membership. The group, which included policy analysts, doctors, and representatives of labor, business, and private health plans, was able to look beyond many differing individual views in order to agree on these fundamental principles. In the end, they agreed that the ways in which health care is delivered—both within Medicare and in the health care system at large—must change. In particular, they feel that the quality of American health care could be improved greatly by educating Americans about how to recognize superior care. Medicare can play an important role in bringing about this transformation.

On behalf of the Trustees of The Century Foundation, I thank the chairs and the members of the task force; the writers of the background papers, Lisa Potetz and Thomas Rice; as well as Leif Wellington Haase and Jacob Hacker, who drafted the report, for all the hard work that produced this important contribution to this ongoing debate.

Richard C. Leone, *PRESIDENT*
The Century Foundation
August 2001

CONTENTS

MEMBERS OF THE TASK FORCE

Richard Ravitch, Task Force Cochair
Principal, Ravitch, Rice and Company, LLC

Shoshanna Sofaer, Task Force Cochair and Executive Director
Robert P. Luciano Professor of Health Care Policy,
Baruch College, CUNY

Robert N. Alpert
Executive Director, UAW Center for Community Health Care Initiatives

Diane Archer
President, Medicare Rights Center

Brian Biles, M.D.
Professor and Chair, Department of Health Services Management
and Policy, George Washington University

Theresa Bischoff
Acting COO, Mount Sinai NYU Health; President, NYU Hospital
Center

Norman Daniels
Goldthwaite Professor of Philosophy, Tufts University

Judith Feder
Dean of Policy Studies, Georgetown University

Note: The organizations and affiliations of task force members are listed for the purposes of identification only. The opinions expressed in this report are solely those of the individual task force members.

Michael E. Gluck
Research Associate Professor, Institute for Health Care Research and Policy, Georgetown University

Marsha Gold
Senior Fellow, Mathematica Policy Research, Inc.

Jacob S. Hacker
Junior Fellow, Harvard University Society of Fellows

Lauren LeRoy
President and CEO, Grantmakers in Health

Maria Lyzen, R.N.
Manager, Medicare Managed Care Plans, General Motors

Marilyn Moon
Senior Fellow, The Urban Institute

James Mortimer
President, Midwest Business Group on Health

Patricia Neuman
Vice President, Henry J. Kaiser Family Foundation

Albert Siu, M.D.
Clifford Spingarn, M.D. Professor of Medicine, The Mount Sinai School of Medicine

Harvey I. Sloane, M.D.
Public Health Director, Eurasian Medical Education Program; Policy Analyst, Project HOPE

Robyn Stone
Executive Director, Institute for the Future of Aging Services; American Association of Homes and Services for the Aging

Daniel B. Wolfson
Former President and CEO, Alliance of Community Health Plans

ACKNOWLEDGMENTS

This report represents two years of deliberations by a group of talented and committed individuals who made time in their extremely busy schedules to struggle toward a meaningful consensus on difficult issues. They were respectful of one another's perspectives and were able and willing both to speak their minds and to change their minds.

In addition to acknowledging the members of the group, who made a difficult task genuinely enjoyable for me, it is clear that our work would not have moved forward and come to a fruitful conclusion without the remarkable support provided by The Century Foundation. Richard C. Leone and Greg Anrig were gracious hosts who kept us focused on the need to produce a document that would be well grounded in the best available evidence and analysis and that would have both immediate and longer-term relevance to discussions of Medicare reform.

Leif Wellington Haase served as our primary staff support for the entire life of the task force. It would be impossible to overestimate his contributions. He brought his native and well-honed analytical and writing skills to bear on what task force members had to say. Leif was backed up, over the course of the project, by the able support first of Benjamin Moodie and then Eelco Slagter. In the last few months, one member of the Task Force, Jacob Hacker, stepped up to the plate to play a far more significant role in drafting (and redrafting, and reredrafting) chapters of this work and in reviewing all the others in considerable depth.

I want to thank The Century Foundation for giving me the opportunity to participate in this enterprise with this group of people. As is always the case for those who, as Jane Austen says, "love to instruct," I learned much more than I contributed.

Shoshanna Sofaer
Task Force Executive Director

REPORT OF THE TASK FORCE

Introduction:
Principles and Summary

In July 2000 Medicare turned thirty-five. The significance of this birthday is open to multiple interpretations. Among experts and the general public, opinions vary about whether the nation's federal health insurance plan for older Americans and the disabled faces a full-blown midlife crisis, deserves thorough reexamination, or rates a mostly clean bill of health.

What is beyond dispute is the gravity of decisions to be made about the program's future. Medicare insures more Americans than any other government health care program, about 39 million people in 2000. It pays for one out of every five dollars spent on health care in the United States. It makes up more than 12 percent of the annual federal budget, and its spending will rise in the future as medical costs and program enrollment increase.

Medicare and Social Security (the federal program for retirement benefits) are far and away the most popular government programs. Ninety-five percent of all Americans believe that it is "very important" or "somewhat important" that Medicare be preserved.[1] Adults aged fifty to sixty-five, the next group that will enter the program, trust it to deliver better access to care, and a higher quality of care, than employer-sponsored group insurance or directly purchased private insurance.[2] Without Medicare, millions of older and disabled Americans would be unable to afford health insurance or to pay for medical care.

The Mission of The Century Foundation Task Force

The debate over Medicare's future has evolved rapidly over the past several years. In 1997, passage of the Balanced Budget Act contributed greatly to ending federal budget deficits, principally by slowing the growth of Medicare payments to hospitals, home health agencies, health care plans, and other medical providers.

This act also established a National Bipartisan Commission on the Future of Medicare to study and make recommendations on the program's long-run financing. When this commission convened, leading members argued that Medicare needed to be reformed swiftly and drastically because of the strain its future spending could place on the federal budget. Projections made by the program's trustees and by the Congressional Budget Office anticipate future shortfalls for Medicare's Hospital Insurance Trust Fund. This reflects the substantial growth in program enrollment that will occur after the baby-boom generation retires and higher medical costs that stem partly from the introduction and diffusion of costly new procedures and therapies. In the end, however, the commission was unable to issue formal recommendations owing to fundamental disagreements between those who wanted to encourage greater participation in Medicare by private health plans in order to reduce spending and those who doubted the potential savings from this approach and feared its impact on beneficiaries.

The Century Foundation's Task Force on Medicare Reform first convened in spring 1999, just before the national commission concluded its work. The members of the task force—policy analysts, physicians, hospital administrators, and representatives of consumer, business, labor, and health plan trade groups—are experts and pratitioners with diverse perspectives on the program.

The task force organized its work around the question, "What do we want Medicare to look like in the future?" To some degree, this effort paralleled that laid out by the cochair of the national Medicare commission, who described the commission's task as "looking at the fundamental question of what we want Medicare to do and what kind of health care system we want for the elderly in our country."[3]

While sharing the concern of the commission's leaders with the adequacy of the program's long-term financing, most members of The Century Foundation's task force did not view Medicare's potential financing difficulties as the primary reform imperative. Some task force members believed that incremental reforms more in keeping with the prior history of changes to Medicare would be prudent, while others favored more significant changes. All agreed, however, that major structural reforms to Medicare should not be made solely on the basis of prognostications of future fiscal doom. Looking beyond issues of Medicare financing, the task force members argued, could open the door to considering reform options—especially those that seem slightly beyond the reach of political possibility—in a new light. This spirit animated the group's deliberations and informs the discussion that follows.

Over the course of five meetings of the full group and a number of discussions among smaller subcommittees of the group, the task force identified four major areas of agreement. The members agreed that:

- Medicare's character as a social insurance program should be preserved;

- the future cost of financing the program is not the only problem that reforms must address;

- the coverage provided by the current program is inadequate; and

- Congress and program administrators should explore ways to improve the quality and value of services that are paid for by Medicare and implement these approaches.

Much of the work of the task force was devoted to refining a set of general principles that would express these areas of agreement in more practical terms and thus bear upon both current and future debates over Medicare reform. These principles are listed below. Each principle refers to a critical element of program design, such as financing, the scope of the benefit package, and consumer choice. Taken together, the principles are intended to respond to the major issues that policymakers will need to consider when proposing comprehensive reforms to Medicare. While the details of proposals change, certain basic approaches to Medicare reform tend to persist. To be sure, there are other issues that large-scale reform would have to take into account, such as Medicare's role in funding medical education and its possible expansion as a payer for long-term care. But the task force felt that these other areas were either more technical in nature or removed from the current policy debate compared to the features of Medicare that are discussed in the principles and rationale.

The remainder of this introduction summarizes the essential points of the full report and relates the principles to these broad areas of agreement. The body of the report explains why these particular principles were chosen, defends their choice, and illustrates how they can be used to judge particular Medicare reform proposals.

PRINCIPLES FOR MEDICARE REFORM OF THE CENTURY FOUNDATION'S TASK FORCE

I.   Medicare should remain a social insurance program that protects older and disabled Americans from the financial burden of health care, that shares the financial risk of serious illness and disability among the millions of Americans who are covered and who will be covered, and that requires contributions from workers and employers.

II. Medicare should continue to be financed in part through general revenues and in part by contributions from workers, employers, and the covered population, but as Medicare's financial needs grow, older and disabled Americans should not shoulder a significantly higher proportion of program expenditures or medical costs.

III. The scope of health care benefits covered under Medicare should be expanded to include elements that are critical to preventing or detecting disease and managing chronic conditions, as well as treating acute illness.

IV. Proposals to reform Medicare should reduce and eliminate, rather than maintain or exacerbate, the disadvantages faced by vulnerable populations within the program.

V.   Medicare should be a responsible steward that works to promote and encourage high quality care and the efficient delivery of medical services.

VI. The process by which people with Medicare choose among alternative health insurance options and products should be made easier: it should clarify important distinctions among different types of health insurance and provide useful and unbiased education, information, and decision support to beneficiaries and those who help them make choices.

VII. Medicare's management and administrative capacities should be adequately funded so that the goals implied by these principles can be carried out effectively in the context of a growing Medicare population.

MEDICARE'S CHARACTER AS A SOCIAL INSURANCE PROGRAM MUST BE PRESERVED (PRINCIPLE I)

The members of the task force strongly felt that any reforms to Medicare should not jeopardize the program's social insurance character. Social insurance offers collective protection against a set of risks that private insurance markets are unlikely to insure against at an affordable cost.[4] In the United States, such programs characteristically involve the payment of a dedicated tax, administration by government or other public authority, and provision of benefits under uniform statutory rules. In Social Security, this benefit is a cash replacement for wage income. In Medicare, it constitutes payment for hospital stays, physicians' services, and other medical services.

All insurance plans pool risk, but social insurance programs like Medicare do so in distinctive ways. As one analyst puts it: "Health insurance, life insurance, disability insurance, and annuities—the principal components of Social Security and Medicare—can be found in the private market. But Social Security and Medicare insure against risks such as living longer than average; not earning a good living; and obtaining access to very specialized care generally or relatively routine care in both poor urban and poor rural areas"[5] Medicare helps protect against the large expenses that can—and do—occur as the prices of medical procedures and other services rise. Since the benefit package is uniform and the premiums for insurance do not rise with age, older, poorer, and sicker Americans get an especially good deal.[6] In addition, Medicare-eligible beneficiaries who are at or near the poverty line may have all or part of their premiums and copayments paid for by Medicaid, the federal/state health program for poor Americans who meet other criteria for eligibility.

Medicare modestly redistributes wealth from better-off to less well-off Americans. Unlike Social Security, there is no income ceiling on the payroll tax that funds the hospital insurance portion of Medicare. General revenues, which fund most of the payments for physicians' services, are more progressive than payroll taxes. Since Medicare relies in part on compulsory payments by current workers, it shares risk among different generations as well. Unlike workers in many other developed nations, American workers under the age of sixty-five contribute to a program for which they typically become eligible only when they reach retirement age. This magnifies the importance of retaining the social compact among different generations that has supported Medicare to date.

MEDICARE'S COSTS ARE HARD TO PREDICT, AND THEIR BURDEN SHOULD BE SHARED FAIRLY (PRINCIPLE II)

What Medicare costs—rather than what the program accomplishes for seniors, the disabled, and their families—has been the principal focus of Congress during much of the program's lifetime. This is not surprising. The steady rise of Medicare expenditures in the 1970s and 1980s exceeded the rate of inflation and contributed to the growth of federal deficits.[7] Demographic and economic projections show a growing population of older, longer-lived Americans and rising medical costs, especially prescription drug costs.

However, placing such a strong emphasis on Medicare's financing and on its expected long-run impact on the federal budget tends to obscure the reality of Medicare's current fiscal situation and the importance of the program's basic aims. For example:

The Fiscal Situation Has Improved. Medicare's financing looks more sturdy than experts predicted several years ago. As recently as 1997, the trustees of the Hospital Insurance Trust Fund warned that this fund could be depleted by 2001. Though projections of near-term trust fund insolvency had not been uncommon, the new numbers helped focus additional attention on the program's financing. The Balanced Budget Act of 1997 has had a more potent effect in reducing Medicare's expenditures than expected, while a strong economy has boosted revenues. In 1999, for the first time, Medicare spending actually decreased by 1.5 percent, compared to a growth rate of slightly more than 4 percent for private health insurance. Thanks to this favorable trend, the Part A Trust Fund is now expected to be in the black through 2029.[8] These developments do not counsel complacency, but they certainly appear to be grounds for deliberate rather than hasty action.

Projections Are Uncertain. The rapid changes from shortfalls (or anticipated shortfalls) to surpluses, in both the federal budget and in the Medicare Trust Fund, point out the uncertainty of projections, especially long-run projections, and the dangers to policymakers of relying too heavily on these estimates. The budget deficit for the 1998 fiscal year, for example, was estimated in 1993 at $357 billion, while the actual figure turned out to be a $69 billion surplus.[9] The 1999 Congressional Budget Office forecast of Medicare spending for the 2000–2007 period was more than $530 billion less than the office had predicted in 1997.[10] To be sure, projections have been known to understate as well as overstate future obligations. But these trends offer a fundamental caution against basing policy changes largely on estimates of future costs.

Changes in various social and economic trends could ease the effect of the baby-boom generation's retirement on taxpayers. Some of these changes are incorporated in official projections, while others are not. The size of the labor force and of the elderly population itself may vary. Reduced disability among the elderly—perhaps accelerated by behavioral changes and new medical treatments at the genetic level—could conceivably lower Medicare and Medicaid costs. And it is worth keeping in mind that the size of the U.S. elderly population relative to most other industrialized nations is still quite small. Because the percentage of Americans over the age of sixty-five will approach the current levels of Germany or Japan only by 2020, the United States will have the advantage of observing how other countries deal with this demographic transition.

The most important—and uncertain—determinant of the sustainability of government programs is the rate of economic growth. Citizens of a nation that grows steadily wealthier can afford to pay higher taxes for social welfare programs while still raising their living standards. One 1999 study, for example, estimated that if U.S. economic growth averages 2.8 percent over the next thirty years (slightly less than the 2.9 percent it has averaged over the past thirty-two years), government spending as a share of GNP will remain constant despite the anticipated demographic changes.[11]

Increased Medicare Spending May Be Worth the Cost. Several recent studies argue that there is a strong connection between the availability of Medicare and the overall improvement in the health of seniors and the disabled over time. In particular, reductions in mortality have been concentrated among the elderly since 1966, in large part thanks to better prevention and treatment of cardiovascular disease.[12] Functional disabilities also have declined among seniors, and new technologies such as artificial joints have improved their quality of life.[13] Depending on how much advances in medicine reduce morbidity and disability for older Americans and how highly society weighs the value of these improvements, higher Medicare spending may in fact be worth the cost.

Trends in public spending on health care also should be gauged by the number of beneficiaries served. Since the number of Medicare beneficiaries is expected to rise substantially after the baby-boom generation (those born between 1946 and 1964) retires, the proportion of overall spending on Medicare is likely to rise in tandem (see Figure 1). If Americans continue to place a high priority on the program's aims, and assuming per capita increases are kept to a reasonable rate of growth, this spending is likely to gain public support.

The Future of Private Plans in Medicare Is Uncertain. The 1997 Balanced Budget Act aimed to increase the number and variety of private health plans, mostly managed care plans, that could contract with Medicare. The establishment of the Medicare+Choice program

---

FIGURE 1. GROWTH IN THE U.S. ELDERLY POPULATION, HISTORIC DATA AND PROJECTIONS

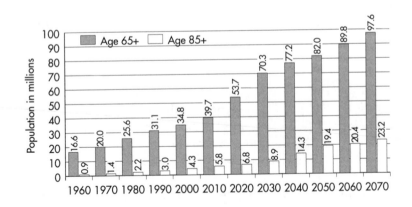

Source: "Growth in the U.S Elderly Population, Historic Data and Projections," U.S. Department of Commerce, Bureau of the Census, available at http://www.census.gov/ipc/prod/97agewcl.pdf, p. 6.

under the BBA was the most important provision of this kind (see Box 1, page 12). Many supporters of the bill regarded the implementation of Medicare+Choice as the first step toward introducing a much broader element of competition in Medicare. Alarmed at the prospects of escalating Medicare expenditures and of new deficits that might crimp investment and stifle future economic growth, these proponents argued that competition among plans would yield quality health care, dismantle an inefficient government bureaucracy, and eventually reduce government spending. A "premium support" proposal under which Medicare beneficiaries would apply an annual government contribution toward the premium of a plan they select is the legislative centerpiece of this competition-based approach to Medicare reform (see Box 2, page 15).

The background paper by Lisa Potetz, a health policy consultant, offers an in-depth analysis of the extent to which the Medicare program should rely on competition among private plans to provide benefits to enrollees. Potetz discusses both the theory and practice behind this managed competition approach. Her paper illustrates the difficulties of using Medicare+Choice as a platform on which to build a superstructure of greater plan competition. Though expected to enroll a rapidly increasing number of beneficiaries, growth in the program has leveled off, and the number of enrolled beneficiaries actually shrank in 2000. Medicare HMO withdrawals from the Medicare+Choice program—either from the program altogether or in certain areas—affected more than 2 million beneficiaries in the three-year period from 1998 to 2000, and many of the newer plan options have not been offered at all. Health plans that dropped Medicare coverage cited too-low payment rates and burdensome regulations, while beneficiaries who had been attracted by the more generous benefit packages saw those benefits shrink. Replacing the current system of payments to plans, which is linked to fee-for-service rates, with one based on competitive pricing, under which a plan's premiums would reflect its bid to cover a basic Medicare benefit package, might result in fairer payments. However, demonstration projects designed to study the feasibility of this approach have been beset by difficulties.[14]

In the early 1990s, large employers enjoyed considerable success paring their expenditures on health care by turning to managed care plans to enroll their employees. Many legislators and policymakers were eager to see if Medicare could do likewise. Recent trends suggest,

BOX 1. MEDICARE FEE-FOR-SERVICE, MANAGED CARE, AND MEDICARE+CHOICE

At its inception, Medicare was set up as a "fee-for-service" program. For most beneficiaries, it remains a fee-for-service arrangement to this day. Beneficiaries choose from any provider who accepts Medicare patients. Medicare reimburses hospitals with a set price for an episode of care determined by a patient's diagnosis, while paying physicians based on a fee schedule.[a] Most physicians "accept assignment," meaning that Medicare's fee is accepted as payment in full for covered procedures and treatments. Some doctors choose to bill patients an additional amount that is limited by law ("balance billing").

Since the early 1970s, and especially after new laws took effect in 1985, Medicare beneficiaries have been permitted to enroll in Medicare managed care plans. In contrast to fee-for-service arrangements, managed care is understood as a system in which health plans construct a network of providers and adopt particular payment and coverage rules. Individuals who join managed care plans typically accept some restrictions on their choice of provider in return for lower premium costs or more health benefits, or both.

Until the mid-1990s, Medicare beneficiaries who chose managed care plans were enrolled almost exclusively in health maintenance organizations (HMOs), the best-known form of managed care. Under this arrangement, plans agree to offer the services covered by the Medicare benefit package in return for a fixed amount per enrollee ("capitation") from the government. If Medicare's payments exceed a plan's profit in its private commercial business, the plan is required to provide additional benefits to enrollees, lower its cost sharing, or return the excess money to the government.

Attracted in large part by the possibility of receiving extra benefits, especially prescription drugs with little or no increase in their premiums, the proportion of Medicare beneficiaries enrolled in managed care grew to 16 percent by 1998. Access to these plans, however, varied considerably for a number of reasons, including Medicare's method of paying them. Medicare pegged the capitation rate for plans at 95 percent of the average cost for a fee-for-service beneficiary in a given county, with some adjustments for the demographics and other characteristics of the payment area. Plans clustered in metropolitan areas where fee-for-service reimbursements were high and physicians were plentiful. At least until the early 1990s, and possibly up to the present, plans attracted beneficiaries who were healthier than the Medicare average, meaning that the government overpaid because of this favorable selection.[b]

Cont. on the next page

Box 1. Medicare Fee-for-Service, Managed Care, and Medicare+Choice (cont.)

The Balanced Budget Act of 1997 (BBA) tried to remedy these flaws by partially uncoupling the managed care payments from local fee-for-service rates, requiring the creation and implementation of a new "risk adjustment" method for paying plans, and establishing a demonstration project for competitive pricing approaches. However, for a variety of reasons, including the effects of reductions in Medicare payments to providers and plans that also were included in the BBA, these policies have not yet begun to achieve their intended results.[c]

The 1997 BBA established the Medicare+Choice program with the intent of expanding the options available to beneficiaries for enrolling in private health plans. The Medicare+Choice program incorporated the existing Medicare managed care plans and allowed new types of managed care plans, such as provider-sponsored plans, to contract with Medicare. It also permitted plans other than the managed care kind to accept Medicare patients, some of which (like private fee-for-service plans) were exempt from regular Medicare payment and coverage rules.

Contrary to expectations, growth in Medicare+Choice has thus far failed to materialize. Few new private plans have decided to contract with Medicare. In fact, faced with rising costs for prescription drugs and other health costs, a number of insurers have withdrawn either completely from the program or from some areas; those that remain have tended to raise their premiums and cost sharing for beneficiaries. At least 934,000 beneficiaries will be affected by Medicare+Choice withdrawals and service reductions in 2001, following 407,000 in 1999 and 327,000 in 2000 who were similarly affected. A majority of these beneficiaries were able to join other HMOs, but others (about 17 percent of those affected in 2001) will have to return to traditional fee-for-service Medicare or to join a Medigap plan, in most cases facing a reduction of benefits and higher out-of-pocket costs.[d]

[a] David G. Smith, *Paying for Medicare: The Politics of Reform* (Hawthorne, N.Y.: Aldine de Gruyter, 1992), is an excellent and detailed study of the origins and nature of Medicare provider payment methods and reforms.

[b] To what extent, if any, this favorable selection into Medicare+Choice plans persists is a subject of considerable debate among health services researchers. Most of the data for studies that have found this effect come from the early 1990s or before; a few studies use sources that date from the mid-1990s. For a summary of the debate and a complete bibliography of the recent literature, see Herbert S. Wong and Fred J. Hellinger, "Conducting Research on the Medicare Market: The Need for Better Data and Methods," *Health Services Research* 36, Part II (April 2001): 291–308. For an argument about the probable convergence of the characteristics of fee-for-service and managed care populations over time, see Mark Pauly and Sean

Cont. on the next page

**BOX 1. MEDICARE FEE-FOR-SERVICE,
MANAGED CARE, AND MEDICARE+CHOICE (CONT.)**

Nicholson, "Adverse Consequences of Adverse Selection," *Journal of Health Politics, Policy and Law* 24, no. 5 (October 1999): 921–29. For earlier findings of favorable selection into Medicare managed care, see R. S. Brown et al., "The Medicare Risk Program for HMOs: Final Summary on Findings from the Evaluation," report submitted to the U.S. Department of Health and Human Services, Mathematica Policy Research, Princeton, N.J., February 1993.
[c] On risk adjustment, see Richard Kronick and Joy de Beyer, *Medicare HMOs: Making Them Work for the Chronically Ill* (Chicago: Health Administration Press, 1998); and Kronick and De Beyer "Risk Adjustment Is Not Enough," Commonwealth Fund, New York, 1997. On competitive pricing, see Len M. Nichols and Robert D. Reischauer, "Who Really Wants Price Competition in Medicare Managed Care?" *Health Affairs* 19, no. 5 (September/October 2000): 30–43.
[d] Marsha Gold, "Trends Reflect Fewer Choices," *Monitoring Medicare+Choice: Fast Facts*, no. 4, Mathematica Policy Research, Princeton, N.J., September 2000.

---

however, that the dissatisfaction of some consumers with managed care is leading insurers to retreat from many of the techniques, such as restricted provider networks, that may have been central to managed care's ability to control costs.[15] The jury is still out on whether managed care can be effective in the long run in keeping down overall health care costs.[16]

MEDICARE'S COVERAGE IS INADEQUATE (PRINCIPLES III AND IV)

The task force believes that Medicare, while highly successful in achieving its primary goals of improving the economic security of the elderly and disabled and their access to care, requires reforms that would make its benefits more comparable to those routinely available in private health insurance plans while encouraging care that reflects new innovations in medicine that can improve the health and quality of life of older Americans.

Medicare's most glaring weakness is its absence of coverage for almost all outpatient prescription drugs. As more medical procedures are performed on an outpatient basis, and as an aging population develops more chronic illnesses, this absence has become more significant. Unlike most private insurance plans, Medicare also lacks "stop-loss" protection that pays for very high medical expenses above a cap. Since Medicare covers only a set number of hospital days per benefit period and over a lifetime, expenses can mount rapidly for the very few beneficiaries who exceed this limit. Likewise, the cost sharing

Box 2. Premium Support

Premium support, a term given to a comprehensive restructuring proposal for Medicare, would involve the payment of a fixed government contribution on behalf of a beneficiary toward the premium of a health plan that contracts with Medicare. A beneficiary would pay the difference between this amount and the cost of the premium of the plan he or she selected.

Modeled on the Federal Employees Health Benefits Program (FEHBP), premium support would replace the traditional fee-for-service Medicare program with a system based on beneficiary choice among competing health plans.[a] The traditional program offers a standard benefit package and identical premiums and establishes prices for thousands of medical procedures. Under a premium support model, the federal sponsor would negotiate with health plans rather than set fees for providers. These plans would construct provider networks and offer different benefit packages with varying premiums (though a minimum benefit package probably would be specified in law). The traditional fee-for-service program would become one of the competing plans and adopt its own premium. Medicare's payment to health plans would be based on the cost of an average premium and adjusted for the characteristics of a plan's enrolled population. The underlying expectation for premium support is that informed Medicare beneficiaries will choose plans that offer the most value, thereby saving money for themselves and for the program as a whole.

A premium support proposal was at the heart of a bill first introduced by Senators John Breaux (D.-La.) and Bill Frist (R.-Tenn) during the 106th Congress [S.1895] and reintroduced in similar form in the 107th Congress [S.357]. (For a fuller description and critique of this proposed reform, see the background paper by Lisa Potetz, "Competition-based Approaches to Medicare Reform," in this volume.)

In his 1999 plan for Medicare reform, President Clinton proposed a "competitive defined benefit" idea.[b] Private health plans would be reimbursed based on the price of their bid on a standard Medicare benefit package including a drug benefit.[c] If beneficiaries selected lower-cost plans, they would pay lower premiums. The government would realize savings as well. The logic of this proposal resembles that of premium support in its intent to stimulate competition among health plans and choice among beneficiaries. It would replace the existing system that links payments to plans to fee-for-service costs in a given area. However, the competitive defined benefit idea, unlike premium support proposals, would not restructure Medicare.

Cont. on the next page

Box 2. Premium Support (Cont.)

It would apply only to existing health plans that contract with Medicare, leaving the traditional fee-for-service program intact. Beneficiaries who chose to remain in this program would pay no more than the Part B premium as specified in statute. Under premium support, on the other hand, they might pay considerably more than this amount depending on how the cost of a fee-for-service arrangement compared over time with that of other competing health plans.

[a] For a full description of the ways in which the idea of premium support evolves from the existing program of health benefits for federal employees, see Mark Merlis, *Medicare Restructuring: The FEHBP Model*, Henry J. Kaiser Family Foundation, Washington, D.C., February 1999. An early statement of the premium support idea may be found in Henry J. Aaron and Robert D. Reischauer, "The Medicare Reform Debate: What Is the Next Step?" *Health Affairs* 14, no. 4 (Winter 1995): 8–30.
[b] See "The President's Plan to Modernize and Strengthen Medicare for the 21st Century," National Economic Council and Domestic Policy Council, July 2, 1999, pp. 8–13.
[c] Initially, this payment would not exceed 96 percent of the cost of Medicare's original fee-for-service payments for the average beneficiary, though plans also would be explicitly subsidized for offering drug coverage.

for physician services and other Part B procedures, generally set at 20 percent of the allowable cost of care, can be a hurdle for lower-income beneficiaries whose income just exceeds the limit under which they can seek assistance from Medicaid.

Medicare's lack of comprehensive coverage means that most beneficiaries either purchase supplemental insurance (Medigap), receive coverage through a previous employer (or a spouse's employer), or obtain additional benefits through HMOs. Just 9 percent of beneficiaries had only Medicare coverage in 1998. But, as Thomas Rice of the UCLA School of Public Health shows in his background paper on supplemental insurance, the availability of these sources of insurance is decreasing, and their cost is increasing rapidly. As these sources of coverage dwindle, the number of Americans favoring a more comprehensive benefit package is likely to rise.

MEDICARE SHOULD ACTIVELY SEEK WAYS TO IMPROVE THE VALUE OF THE SERVICES IT PAYS FOR (PRINCIPLES V, VI, AND VII)

Members of the task force felt that the value of the medical services that Medicare pays for should be and could be improved. Concerns about medical errors, worries about the high cost of care, better evidence about the effectiveness of treatments in yielding desired outcomes, and greater awareness of how financial incentives affect the delivery of health care have combined to bring this issue to the fore. For example, a recent Institute of Medicine report, *Crossing the Quality Chasm: A New Health System for the 21st Century*, criticized the "highly fragmented delivery system" that "does not, as a whole, make the best use of its resources" and expressed regret at "the absence of real progress toward restructuring health care systems to address both quality and cost concerns."[17]

The task force felt that Medicare could play a major role in this potential revamping of the U.S. health system while noting that it needs to move cautiously because of its special responsibilities as a publicly accountable program and for other reasons of custom and statute.[18] Some ways the program might encourage greater value in the delivery of care could involve:

- taking steps toward improving the quality of care delivered by providers and plans that contract with Medicare and toward better care in the medical system as a whole (Principle V);

- adopting methods for developing and disseminating information about providers and plans so that Medicare beneficiaries can make informed and meaningful choices about their coverage (Principle VI); and

- dedicating more resources to the program's management (Principle VII).

Much effort in quality improvement revolves around applying clinical evidence to everyday medical procedures with the aim of reducing unneeded or potentially harmful care and steering resources toward necessary care. (The wide difference in per capita spending on Medicare patients in different parts of the United States, even after attempts to adjust for the characteristics of the populations served, is one piece of evidence that leads researchers to believe that spending on health care does not necessarily correlate with health gains.[19]) The Health Care Financing Administration (HCFA), the federal agency that runs Medicare,[20] has expanded its existing quality assurance programs to monitor how well health plans and some providers adhere to "process" measures of quality—carrying out clinical interventions that research shows will produce better health outcomes, such as administering beta blockers to heart attack victims. More aggressive ways of using Medicare's market power to improve quality might involve contracting selectively with providers who met or exceeded various predetermined performance measures. Assuming these measures accurately reflect the underlying data and that this type of contracting does not unduly affect access to care, they are worth considering.

Measures to enhance quality in Medicare or to introduce more choice for beneficiaries depend fundamentally on enrollees becoming more knowledgeable about the real distinctions between different kinds of health insurance products, such as original Medicare, health maintenance organizations, and Medigap, as well as on the development of "user-friendly" data. This is challenging in part because Medicare beneficiaries are a diverse group. In particular, those with cognitive and physical impairments, or whose first language is not English, vary in their capacity for understanding the program. Studies also show that beneficiaries as a group have a sketchy understanding not only of new and potential options under Medicare but of traditional Medicare as well. HCFA, which formerly dealt almost exclusively with providers, has been expanding its efforts both to develop and to disseminate useful comparative data for beneficiaries. For this effort to be successful, "information intermediaries," especially those based in organizations that assist seniors and people with disablities, will need to evolve.

Compared to private insurers, Medicare features low administrative costs as a percentage of benefits paid (around 1–2 percent annually), as opposed to a much higher percentage (9.5 percent per year according to one estimate[21]) in the private sector. To the extent that this reflects maintaining a lower disenrollment rate among the covered population and not having to incur marketing costs, it is advantageous. However, the amount spent on administration may not be optimal given the rise in program spending, complexity, and enrollment. HCFA has been charged with implementing and overseeing a large number of new regulations, especially those included in the Balanced Budget Act of 1997 and in subsequent bills that amended it. Dedicating more resources to program management is essential to expanding the capacity of administrators both to streamline and to carry out the regulations that are on the books—both in terms of enforcement and in terms of offering adequate support to providers, plans, and beneficiaries.

Medicare is obligated to those it covers to ensure that treatments are safe and of high quality. It also is accountable to the taxpayers and beneficiaries who pay the program's bills. Focusing on value raises hopes for a modus vivendi between the two imperatives that generally drive reform proposals: the need for fiscal restraint and the need for a more comprehensive benefit package and a more rational payment system.

A wealth of excellent books and reports explains how to navigate Medicare, laying out its basic rules and coverage policies. First-rate histories of the program exist. Policy analyses (and policy nostrums) are legion. With few exceptions, however, the debate lacks an accessible guide that develops a set of principles through which a variety of reform proposals can be evaluated while identifying the context for both principles and policies. This task force report strives to fill that gap.

1.

SOCIAL INSURANCE

*Principle I. Medicare should remain a social insurance pro-
gram that protects older and disabled Americans from the
financial burden of health care, that shares the financial risks
of serious illness and disability among the millions of
Americans who are covered and who will be covered, and that
requires contributions from workers and employers.*

Social insurance protects against major threats to individual and
family income to which most citizens are vulnerable. These risks
include losing a job, retiring from the workforce, becoming disabled,
and confronting a costly sickness or accident.[1]

Although private insurance and social insurance share common
elements, they are not the same.[2] Individuals and families can purchase private policies that guard against some (but not all) of the common risks that social insurance programs cover. Yet social insurance
departs from conventional private insurance in two important respects:

1. Social insurance is inclusive in coverage and financing, spread-
    ing risks across the population, and requiring contributions from
    all or most citizens. This in turn means that the decision to
    obtain and contribute to social insurance protection is collec-
    tively governed, not simply an individual choice.

2. To ensure broad participation and provide security to the most vul-
    nerable, social insurance is offered on terms that are similar for
    everyone, regardless of risk or income. These terms are especially

favorable to higher-risk groups and lower-income families and individuals, for whom "premiums" are typically more affordable and benefits typically more generous than those they could obtain in the private market.

Medicare embodies these two defining features of social insurance. It provides protection against potentially devastating risks, and it offers coverage on terms favorable to high-risk and low-income citizens. Whatever changes are made to Medicare, these bedrock features of the program should be preserved and strengthened.

MEDICARE AS SOCIAL INSURANCE

Medicare is an inclusive program. It requires a broad base of contributions and offers benefits to all contributors who have met a minimum threshold of eligibility (see Table 1). Employers and most workers each pay half of a mandatory payroll tax of 2.9 percent to fund the Hospital Insurance (Part A) component of Medicare.[3] Although Supplementary Medical Insurance (Part B) is not paid for through earmarked contributions, 75 percent of the cost of the program is financed by general tax revenues, with the other quarter coming out of premiums paid by or on behalf of people in Medicare. In both parts of the program, therefore, the risks of medical costs are spread beyond the immediate beneficiaries to virtually all working Americans.

Just as important, almost all these Americans will in turn become eligible for Medicare themselves. Citizens can automatically receive hospital insurance coverage when they reach the age of sixty-five. Coverage for physicians' services is voluntary, but virtually all of those who qualify opt to sign up because the premiums are so low given the value of the coverage.[4] In addition, unlike health insurance purchased individually in the private market, Medicare is available regardless of current or previous health status. Because premiums are low and coverage is available to all, Medicare offers protection that is especially valuable to older, sicker, and poorer Americans.

Medicare's inclusiveness serves two major goals that are central to social insurance. The first is to maintain a popular program in which all citizens feel they have a stake. In requiring widely distributed contributions, Medicare creates a claim of earned right to benefits. At the same time, it provides especially valuable protection to the poor

TABLE 1. MEDICARE'S RULES AND BENEFITS

MEDICARE HOSPITAL INSURANCE (PART A) FOR 2001

SERVICES	BENEFIT	PATIENT PAYS	MEDICARE PAYS
Hospitalization: Semiprivate room and board, general nursing, and other hospital services and supplies	First 60 days 61st to 90th day 91st to 150th day[a] Beyond 150 days	Up to $792 $198 a day $396 a day All costs	Costs above $792 Costs above $198 a day Costs above $396 a day Nothing
Skilled Nursing Facility Care: Directly following or within 60 days of a hospital stay: semiprivate room and board, skilled nursing and rehabilitative services, and other services and supplies (after a 3-day hospital stay).	First 20 days 21st to 100th day Beyond 100 days	Nothing $99 a day All costs	All approved costs Costs above $97 Nothing
Home Health Care: Part-time or intermittent skilled care, home health aide services, durable medical equipment and supplies, and other services.	Unlimited as long as requirements are met for home health care benefits	Nothing for services; 20 percent for durable medical equipment	All approved costs for services; 80 percent for equipment
Hospice Care: Pain relief, symptom management, and support services for the terminally ill.	For as long as doctor certifies need	Limited cost sharing for outpatient drugs and inpatient palliative care	All but limited costs for outpatient drugs and inpatient palliative care

Cont. on the next page

TABLE 1. MEDICARE'S RULES AND BENEFITS, CONT.

MEDICARE SUPPLEMENTARY MEDICAL INSURANCE (PART B) FOR 2001

SERVICES	PATIENT PAYS	MEDICARE PAYS
All Part B services	Monthly premium of $50 and $100 annual deductible	
Physician and other services[b]	20 percent	80 percent
Outpatient medical and surgical services and supplies	20 percent	80 percent
Outpatient mental health services	50 percent for most services	50 percent for most services
Clinical laboratory services	Nothing	All approved costs
Preventive services	20 percent of most services; none for pap smears, pelvic examinations, and flu shots	80 percent for most services; all for pap smears, pelvic examinations, and flu shots
Outpatient hospital service	Coinsurance or fixed copayment	Remainder of the costs
Other services and equipment: physical, speech, and occupational therapy and durable medical equipment (such as oxygen cylinders)	20 percent for each course of physical or occupational therapy; 20 percent of durable medical equipment expenses	80 percent for therapy; 80 percent of durable medical equipment costs

[a] The 91st to 150th days shown in the chart constitute a lifetime reserve of 60 days, which may be used only once. For each lifetime reserve day, Medicare pays all covered costs except for a daily coinsurance of $396.
[b] These rates apply to "participating physicians," who agree to accept Medicare's fee schedule for all services. Nonparticipating physicians can charge patients up to 15 percent more than the standard rate.

Source: Medicare and You Handbook, Health Care Financing Administration, 2001.

FIGURE 2. INCOME DISTRIBUTION OF THE POPULATION
AGE SIXTY-FIVE AND OLDER, 1998

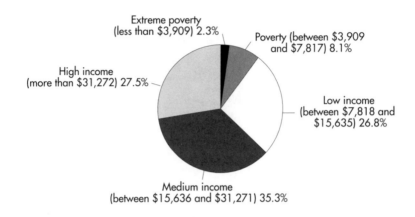

Extreme poverty
(less than $3,909) 2.3%

Poverty (between $3,909
and $7,817) 8.1%

High income
(more than $31,272) 27.5%

Low income
(between $7,818 and
$15,635) 26.8%

Medium income
(between $15,636 and $31,271) 35.3%

Note: Incomes listed here are for one person age sixty-five or over.
Source: Federal Interagency Forum on Aging-Related Statistics, "Older Americans 2000: Key Indicators of Well-being," Current Population Survey data, available at http://www.agingstats.gov/chartbook2000/default.htm, Table 7.

and vulnerable within a common framework into which wealthier and healthier Americans also contribute and from which they also benefit. Medicare is thus a broad-based social contract stretching across income, risk groups, generations, and classes (see Figure 2).[5]

Despite the fierce political debate over Medicare, the foundation of popular support for the program is both deep and wide. In a 1998 poll, for example, 95 percent of Americans agreed that it is important for "Medicare [to be] preserved as a health care program for all people when they retire"(see Figure 3, page 26).[6] Although older Americans are slightly more supportive than the young, almost all groups of Americans oppose reductions in future Medicare spending unless necessary to secure the long-term future of the program.[7] Americans of all generations also say they do not want Medicare's books to be balanced on the backs of the elderly. A 1997 poll, for instance, found citizens of all ages to be overwhelmingly against making the elderly pay a larger share of Medicare costs.[8]

FIGURE 3. HOW IMPORTANT DO AMERICANS CONSIDER THE PRESERVATION OF A HEALTH CARE PROGRAM FOR ALL PEOPLE WHEN THEY RETIRE? (SURVEY CONDUCTED AUGUST–SEPTEMBER 1998)

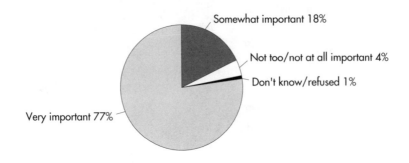

Somewhat important 18%

Not too/not at all important 4%

Don't know/refused 1%

Very important 77%

Source: National Survey on Medicare, Henry J. Kaiser Family Foundation/Harvard School of Public Health, Washington, D.C., October 20, 1998, Chart no.1, available at http://www.kff.org/content/archive/1442/reform_cp.pdf.

The second major goal of Medicare's inclusiveness is to spread the financial risks of medical costs. Because the costs of health care are distributed widely, expensive illnesses suffered by a few individuals are unlikely to drive up the premiums of others. And because both high- and low-risk groups are protected within a common framework, those with higher expected costs are not subject to ruinous expenses or discriminated against on the basis of health. Indeed, by requiring contributions and by drawing on general revenues, Medicare spreads the financial risk of medical care not just across the pool of present beneficiaries but also across generations and over each individual's life span.

This wide spreading of risk is critical because all health insurance programs, public or private, face the problem of "adverse selection"— the tendency for insurance to attract higher-risk groups.[9] Avoiding adverse selection is especially vital if Medicare is to achieve its aim of increasing the security of older Americans. As a group, the elderly suffer from more chronic illnesses and are more prone to sickness or injury than are younger people. Historically, private insurers have been reluctant to offer coverage to the elderly.[10] Moreover, although older Americans are better off than they were just thirty years ago, many could not afford high insurance premiums even if private options were available.

People under the age of sixty-five with long-term disabilities are another high-risk group who would face extremely high premiums or would be unable to obtain health insurance outright without their current access to Medicare. Since 1975, the rate of growth of disabled Americans enrolled in Medicare has been rising faster than that of the elderly.[11] As a group, this population is not well-off: almost 85 percent of the roughly 6 million disabled Medicare beneficiaries in 1995 reported annual incomes of less than $25,000.[12]

The experience of "Medigap" supplemental insurance plans, as described in the accompanying background paper by Thomas Rice, suggests how serious adverse selection in the over-sixty-five market can become. Medicare beneficiaries who choose Medigap plans that offer prescription drug coverage tend to have a greater need for such drugs and to be sicker than the average beneficiary. As a result, the premiums for these policies are extremely high.

Significant features of Medicare guard against adverse selection. In particular, automatic enrollment in Medicare Part A greatly expands the risk pool, as do the highly attractive terms of voluntary enrollment in Part B. Since a sizable proportion of older Americans uses little or no medical care in any given year, the enrollment of nearly all seniors in these two parts of the program cushions the costs of the minority who experience very high expenses.[13] In 1996, for example, the 10 percent of beneficiaries who incurred the highest medical costs had average reimbursements of $31,680 per capita, compared with $1,675 per capita for the remaining 90 percent.[14]

Because of these risk-pooling features, Medicare has had considerable success in protecting against the financial risk of incurring large medical expenditures—its fundamental goal.[15] By absorbing more than half of beneficiaries' medical costs, the program makes a critical contribution to the financial well-being of older Americans and people with disabilities. Before the advent of Medicare, senior citizens commonly lacked insurance, and existing insurance covered only a small fraction of hospital expenses.[16] Medicare immediately improved access to health care for seniors and virtually eliminated differences in access to hospitals based on income. In 1965, before the enactment of Medicare, the rate of hospital use was 30 percent higher among the most affluent older Americans than among the least affluent. By 1967, this gap had closed, and it has remained closed since—even as per day hospital costs have more than tripled.[17] Although ethnic, racial, and geographic disparities in access continue to exist, as discussed elsewhere in the report, they are significantly less severe among Medicare beneficiaries than among Americans as a whole.

The social compact that supports Medicare also extends across generations: Medicare frees many younger and middle-age Americans from worries about how to pay for their aging parents and relatives and, at the same time, helps them feel more secure about their own retirement years. For this reason, it is a mistake to see the debate over Medicare as inevitably pitting generations against each other in a zero-sum struggle of "us" versus "them." Not only do younger Americans benefit from Medicare when a parent or close relative is provided financial and health security; they also benefit when the program to which they contribute is preserved for their own retirement years. All Americans, young and old, have an interest in a secure and dynamic Medicare program.

Finally, like other social insurance programs, Medicare also helps insure against a number of risks for which it is difficult to find coverage in private markets. These include *longevity risk*, the possibility that individuals will outlive their savings; *inflation risk*, the chance that savings will be eroded by rising prices; *market risk*, the danger that assets intended to support retirement will decline in value or grow more slowly than average; and *medical risk*, the likelihood that the norms of appropriate treatment will change over time.[18] Even the most prudent, savings-conscious individual will find it hard to plan effectively in the face of these risks since they are highly unpredictable and play out over a long time. By the same token, many people left to their own devices would fail to make any provision against these risks, failing to recognize their own vulnerability or hoping that others would come to their rescue if necessary. The sometimes dire situation faced by those who need institutional or in-home custodial care for long periods provides a clear illustration of what happens when these sort of difficult-to-insure risks are not protected against.

Of course, Medicare does not protect against all the risks that may arise from the financial burden of illness. From the beneficiary's perspective, it sets no upper bound on costs that may arise from an unusually prolonged hospital stay or on the total cost of coinsurance for most Part B procedures and services. As noted in the introduction, the program does not cover most outpatient prescription drug purchases and excludes a number of preventive services, as well as coverage for custodial long-term care. The incompleteness of Medicare coverage has fostered the development of a secondary market for individually purchased supplemental (Medigap) insurance. It also has encouraged the inclusion of supplemental medical coverage in many retirees' benefit packages and has left Medicaid carrying much of the growing expense of long-term care for older Americans of modest means.

These shortcomings in Medicare coverage do not, however, indicate that the program has failed to provide valuable risk protection. Rather, as upcoming sections of this report will discuss, the incomplete areas of Medicare coverage mainly suggest that Medicare's protection has not fully responded to the rapidly rising cost of medical care, changes in medical technology and practice, and declines in the generosity of supplemental coverage enjoyed by many retirees. Even with these gaps in coverage, Medicare provides broad social insurance protection that is extremely valuable to all Americans. Whether it will continue to uphold the promise of social insurance will depend in part on what changes are made to the program in the years ahead.

THE POTENTIAL IMPACT OF PROPOSED REFORMS

Much of the debate over Medicare has concerned financing—specifically, how the nation will absorb rising medical costs and pay for the growing number of older Americans who will enroll in the program in the coming decades. Yet proposals to restructure Medicare will affect not just how much the program spends but also the extent to which it spreads risks and offers affordable coverage to the most vulnerable. If Medicare is to remain a social insurance program that enjoys wide support, policymakers must pay close attention to the possible effects of proposed reforms on the program's ability to offer inclusive coverage on terms favorable to all citizens.

For example, raising the eligibility age for Medicare has been a widely discussed option for reducing the program's expenses.[19] Yet such a change would gravely affect Medicare's social insurance character. As already discussed, Medicare must be understood in part as a response to the intrinsic difficulties that private insurance markets confront in insuring older and disabled Americans, who are beset by both high and highly concentrated medical costs, frequently live on limited incomes, and are generally unable to obtain group coverage through employment.[20] Raising the eligibility age would do nothing to address these underlying sources of health insecurity. It would simply shift a portion of Medicare costs from public budgets onto the newly ineligible population (and, for those with emloyment-based insurance, their employers), and the greatest burden by far would be borne by those with the fewest resources and greatest need for medical coverage.[21] Furthermore, moving younger and generally healthier Americans out of the common risk pool would undercut Medicare's ability to offset the higher costs of older beneficiaries. Thus, raising the eligibility age would restrict the scope of Medicare's social insurance promise in a manner that is difficult to defend on the grounds of equity or efficiency.

Similarly, two other proposed reforms—*medical savings accounts* and *individual savings accounts* (see Box 3)—are clearly at odds with the social insurance philosophy and practices that Medicare currently embodies. Each would create an alternative to traditional Medicare that would be particularly attractive to healthier and wealthier senior citizens, thus worsening the financial situation of the program as a whole and its ability to spread risk beyond the costliest beneficiaries. Because individual savings accounts proposals would also allow *working* Americans to divert their Medicare contributions into private accounts to be used in retirement, their effect on Medicare's broad-based contribution system would be particularly severe. Both proposed reforms also could undercut the widespread political support for Medicare by fracturing the beneficiary population into distinct groups with differing stakes in the program.

Other leading reform proposals would have less certain and more complicated effects but could nonetheless significantly affect Medicare's standing as social insurance. This is particularly true of so-called *premium support* proposals—which, as Box 2 describes and the background paper by Lisa Potetz analyzes in more detail, would comprehensively restructure Medicare to encourage competition between private health plans and the traditional program. Premium support proposals would fundamentally change the way in which Medicare contracts with private health plans, requiring that the original fee-for-service program and private plans submit price bids while structuring the level of premiums to make Medicare enrollees more sensitive to the cost differences among alternative insurance options.

The premium support idea was the centerpiece of the proposed reforms discussed but not formally recommended by the members of the National Bipartisan Commission on the Future of Medicare.[22] It received its most complete legislative embodiment in a bill introduced

Box 3. Medical Savings Accounts and Individual Accounts

Medicare Medical Savings Accounts

The Medicare Medical Savings Account, one of the options under the Medicare+Choice program, combines a Medical Savings Account (MSA) and a high-deductible health insurance policy. Medicare pays the premium for the policy and makes a contribution to a beneficiary's MSA. The beneficiary uses the money in the MSA to pay for medical services. This money also may be used to pay for medical services not ordinarily covered under Medicare, as well as for certain kinds of nonmedical expenses. Beneficiaries accept the risk of having to pay for all medical expenses once the MSA is depleted and the health insurance policy's deductible has not yet been met. Once the beneficiary has incurred medical costs that exceed the deductible, the policy bears all these costs, including cost sharing. As of spring 2001, no organization had signed a contract to offer a Medicare MSA plan.[a]

Individual Medicare Savings Accounts

Proposals for individual Medicare savings accounts share the basic idea of Americans accumulating a personal retirement account for health care during their working lifetime. They would use this tax-advantaged account, which would be created by a mandatory flat tax on wages, to purchase health insurance during their retirement. The expectation is that individual investors can capture the historically high returns associated with corporate equities and bonds (compared to the U.S. Treasury bills that the Medicare trust funds hold) and exercise greater discretion, as with an MSA, about which health benefits they wish to purchase.

All proposals for individual accounts would trade off the prospect of lower returns in the current collective system of Medicare financing for a higher degree of individual risk of encountering untimely market downturns or unpredictable health care inflation after retirement. These proposals differ substantially in the degree to which they would partially socialize risks. Some would pool the earnings of members of each age cohort to remit an equal annual contribution,[b] while others would make no adjustment of this kind. Some proposals would place limits on permissible investments, seeking to limit the risk of bad decisions, while others would give investors freer rein.[c]

[a] For a more complete description of MSAs in Medicare, see Medicare Payment Advisory Commission, *Medical Savings Accounts and the Medicare Program*, November 2000.
[b] Phil Gramm, Andrew J. Rettenmaier, and Thomas R. Saving, "Medicare Policy for Future Generations: A Search for a Permanent Solution," *New England Journal of Medicine* 338, no. 18 (April 30, 1998): 1307–11.
[c] Deborah J. Chollet, "Individualizing Medicare," Medicare Brief no. 3, National Academy of Social Insurance, Washington, D.C., May 1999, upon which this summary is based, offers a thorough review of the features of these proposals and their possible ramifications.

in 1999 by Senators John Breaux (the chair of the commission) and Bill Frist. In 2000, Senators Breaux and Frist introduced a scaled-down version of their earlier legislation (known as "Breaux-Frist 2000"), billing it as an achievable first step toward more substantial reform. Both pieces of legislation were reintroduced by the two senators in February 2001.

At the heart of the premium support design is a significant change in Medicare as social insurance. Currently, the overwhelming majority of Medicare beneficiaries receive the basic benefits through a common framework, the original Medicare program. Although roughly one out of every seven beneficiaries obtains coverage through private health plans that contract with Medicare, the effects of these choices on the rest of the beneficiary population are inherently limited because all beneficiaries pay the same basic premium regardless of whether they enroll in original Medicare or a private health plan.

Under a premium support proposal, this would not necessarily be the case. Premiums for private plans and for original Medicare would be set through a competitive bidding process, and the amount that individuals would pay for coverage would vary according to the plan that they chose. If more healthy beneficiaries clustered in lower-cost private plans while sicker beneficiaries joined more expensive private plans or stayed in the traditional fee-for-service plan, significant differences could arise in the premiums that beneficiaries paid. Plans with high premiums (including, most likely, original Medicare) could become inherently unstable as healthier beneficiaries continued to migrate to lower-cost plans, further driving up premiums for those who remained.[23]

Preventing this outcome would depend on the promulgation of extensive rules governing plan practices, benefit packages, and marketing techniques, as well as on the creation of a sophisticated and effective risk-adjustment mechanism. The more sensitive this adjustment mechanism, the more appropriate the payments would be. Unfortunately, however, risk-adjustment techniques are not yet very accurate and, indeed, may never attain the necessary precision.[24] Moreover, recent efforts to increase the information available to Medicare beneficiaries—pursued alongside the push to develop better methods of risk-adjustment—may actually worsen the problem of adverse selection by encouraging beneficiaries to self-segregate themselves into insurance plans that cater to patients in similar health.[25]

These concerns about the premium-support design would not apply with equal force to Breaux-Frist 2000, which would hold Medicare premiums steady relative to current law but would offer rebates to beneficiaries who enrolled in lower-cost private plans while charging higher rates to those who enrolled in higher-cost private plans. (Former President Clinton offered a similar proposal in 1999.) In effect, this scaled-down approach would protect beneficiaries of the original Medicare program from the premium increases that might result if private plans were more efficient or attracted healthier patients. Yet, even in the absence of higher premiums for original Medicare, lower-income beneficiaries might still feel financially pressured to join private plans to obtain a refund or broader benefits. These revised designs forfeit much of the budgetary reward promised by proponents of the premium support approach because the overwhelming majority of the cost savings that older and disabled Americans might realize by joining less expensive plans would accrue to them in the form of rebates rather than to the Medicare program. This suggests that the prevention of risk segmentation and the protection of vulnerable patients—essential for the preservation of social insurance—are to some extent in tension with the cost-containment goals of competitive pricing.

The future effects of these and other leading reform proposals are inherently uncertain. Nonetheless, as the foregoing examples suggest, this uncertainty should not obscure the essential fact that Medicare's social insurance status is at stake in the debate over reform. Preserving the social insurance features of the program will require that America's leaders recognize the value of Medicare's inclusive risk protection and consider carefully the potential threats to it posed by alternative proposals for reform.

2.

FINANCING

Principle II. Medicare should continue to be financed in part through general revenues and in part by contributions from workers, employers, and the covered population, but as Medicare's financial needs grow, older and disabled Americans should not shoulder a significantly higher proportion of program expenditures or medical costs.

Of all the contested political issues that surround Medicare, the future financial standing of the program has received the most attention (see Figure 4, page 36). Warnings of looming insolvency made by the program's trustees and Congressional Budget Office analysts have prompted a series of legislative proposals to restructure the program, and budgetary savings have been the primary motive behind nearly every major change to Medicare over the past two decades. Thanks to robust economic growth and a dramatic stabilization of Medicare spending, the most recent Medicare trustees' report offers a substantially more rosy forecast of the program's finances than was accepted just a few years ago (see Figure 5, page 36). This has not, however, altered the widespread perception that Medicare is fiscally unsustainable without major reform, in part because long-term financing projections remain problematic.[1]

The focus on Medicare's financial standing has had positive and negative effects. On the positive side, it has motivated the search for more effective cost-control techniques while reminding politicians and voters that Medicare has costs as well as benefits. A central premise of this task force report, however, is that the focus on future Medicare spending also can distort the range and nature of reform options considered (see Box 4, page 37, and Figure 6, page 38). Rather

FIGURE 4. MEDICARE INCOME AND EXPENDITURES AS A PERCENTAGE OF GDP, HISTORICAL DATA, AND PROJECTIONS

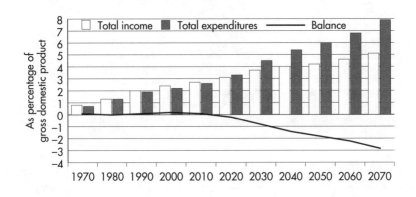

Source: Annual Report of the Board of Trustees of the Federal Hospital Insurance Trust Fund, 2001, Appendix B, Table III B-2.

FIGURE 5. HISTORICAL PROJECTIONS OF HI TRUST FUND INSOLVENCY, 1990–2001

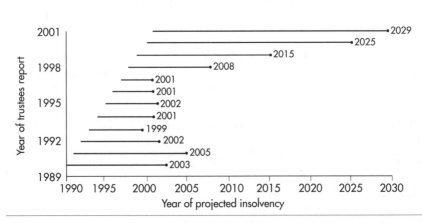

Sources: U.S. Congress, House, Committee on Ways and Means, *2000 Green Book* (Washington, D.C.: U.S. Government Printing Office, 2000), Table 2-9. Data for 2001 comes from the *Annual Report of the Board of Trustees of the Federal Hospital Insurance Trust Fund.*

Box 4. Projecting Medicare Expenditures

Forecasts of Medicare spending growth depend on uncertain projections of medical costs, demographic change, and economic growth. They rest on baseline assumptions—for example, that legislation will remain unchanged for the next thirty years—that are unrealistic by necessity. Projections only provide partial policy guidance: they can suggest the magnitude of new costs that will emerge but not whether they are manageable or justifiable. Cost projections can and should inform policy choices, but they cannot and should not dictate them.[a]

Despite the inherent uncertainty of Medicare forecasts (see Figure 6, page 38), Medicare spending is virtually certain to increase in the coming decades, whether measured as a share of the economy or on an inflation-adjusted per capita basis. First, the proportion of the population that will be enrolled in Medicare is slated to grow dramatically. After rising at a rate of about 1 percent annually between 2000 to 2010, the number of Americans aged sixty-five and over is expected to increase by 3 percent a year from 2010 to 2030. According to the Congressional Budget Office (CBO), the percentage of the population enrolled in Medicare will increase from 13.6 percent in 1995 to 15.2 percent in 2010, to 22 percent in 2030, and to nearly 25 percent in 2070. Rising numbers of beneficiaries translate into rising shares of the national economic product devoted to Medicare, even if costs per beneficiary do not grow faster than the economy itself.

Second, Medicare spending per beneficiary is likely to grow at least modestly faster than the economy as a whole. Historically, increases in national spending on medical services have outpaced both general price inflation and economic growth. Currently, Medicare expenses are growing more slowly than private insurance costs, after a half-decade in which the reverse was true. (Indeed, recent estimates suggest that Medicare spending actually *dropped* in 2000.) Over the long term, however, Medicare's cost path is unlikely to depart too radically from that of private insurance expenditures because both are driven by underlying changes in medical technology, practice, and delivery.

[a] See Joseph White, "Understanding Long-Term Medicare Cost Estimates," white paper, The Century Foundation, New York, 1999.

FIGURE 6. COMPARISON OF ACTUAL HI TRUST FUND EXPERIENCE
WITH ESTIMATES, 1967–93, ABSOLUTE AMOUNTS IN BILLIONS
OF 1993 DOLLARS (1-, 2-, AND 3-YEAR PROJECTIONS)

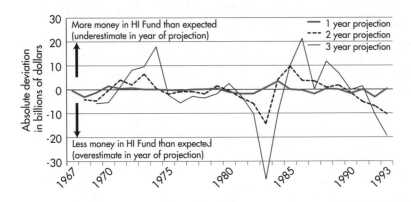

Source: Annual reports of the Board of Trustees of the Federal Old-Age and Survivors Insurance and Disablity Insurance Trust Funds, 1967–1994, available at http://www.ssa.gov/history/reports/trust/trustreports.html.

than ask what Medicare *should* do in the new century, participants in the debate too often begin by asking what Medicare *can afford to do* given the program's past and projected fiscal difficulties. This framing of the issue not only tilts the debate in favor of certain policy choices, it also obscures a larger and more important question: To what extent are Medicare's social insurance commitments worth preserving despite the higher price tag that the program will almost certainly carry in the future?

FINANCING MEDICARE NOW AND IN THE FUTURE

Largely because of the circumstances of its birth, Medicare has a hybrid financing structure that distinguishes it from Social Security's pure contributory framework. The Hospital Insurance (Part A) component of Medicare is financed predominantly from earmarked payroll taxes ($144.4 billion in calendar year 2000, or 86.4 percent of total Hospital Insurance Trust Fund income), as well as from interest on the trust fund and a portion of a tax on Social Security benefits for higher-income beneficiaries.[2] For Supplementary Medical Insurance

(Part B), however, roughly three-quarters of the program's funding comes from general revenues.[3] The other quarter of the program's income comes from premiums paid by or on behalf of current beneficiaries—a percentage that was fixed in law through a provision of the 1997 Balanced Budget Act (see Figure 7, page 40).

Because Medicare is not financed solely by earmarked contributions, the effect of changing demographics on the program is comparatively less pronounced than it is with regard to Social Security. Medicare's financing does not simply transfer a portion of labor market income from current workers to the retired. It also draws income from beneficiaries themselves and from general revenues raised through a range of taxes, not just payroll levies. This pluralism means that Medicare has a number of sources of financing that it could tap in the future besides payroll taxes and that the program would not be departing from historical precedent by relying more heavily on general revenues in the coming decades (although infusing the Part A trust fund with general revenues would be a major departure).

The multiple sources of Medicare financing are somewhat obscured in present debates by the continuing concern with the fiscal solvency of the Part A portion, which is based on a contributory trust fund financed by payroll taxes.[4] Although the trust fund provides a valuable reminder of the link between workers' contributions and benefits, its fiscal standing should not be the sole, or even predominant, criterion used in evaluating Medicare spending. In the first place, Medicare Part B is growing faster than Part A and is likely to be larger than Part A within the next two decades. Unlike the Hospital Insurance Trust Fund, the Part B trust fund cannot ordinarily become insolvent because it is authorized to draw funds as needed from beneficiary premiums and general tax revenues. Moreover, as the population ages and fewer contributors support more beneficiaries, it will necessarily become more difficult to finance Part A benefits through the trust fund alone, even if costs are effectively restrained (see Figure 8, page 41). As a consequence, political leaders will be forced to consider whether the trust fund should be permanently bolstered through increases in payroll contribution rates, the infusion of general revenues, or new beneficiary payments.

The primary means by which Medicare has financed increased spending in the past have been increased reliance on general revenues and, to a lesser extent, increases in Part A contribution rates

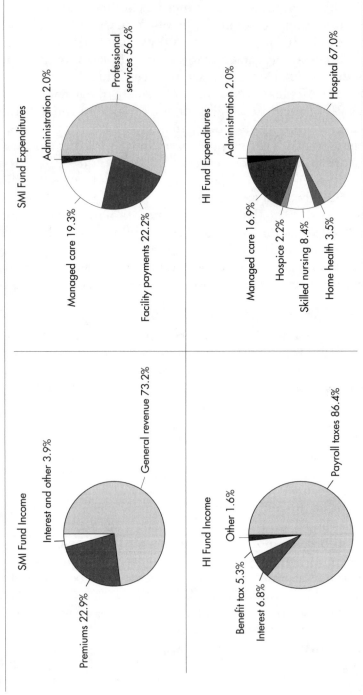

Figure 7. HI and SMI Fund Income and Expenditures, 2000

SMI Fund Income

Interest and other 3.9%

Premiums 22.9%

General revenue 73.2%

SMI Fund Expenditures

Administration 2.0%

Professional services 56.6%

Managed care 19.3%

Facility payments 22.2%

HI Fund Income

Other 1.6%

Benefit tax 5.3%

Interest 6.8%

Payroll taxes 86.4%

HI Fund Expenditures

Administration 2.0%

Hospital 67.0%

Managed care 16.9%

Hospice 2.2%

Skilled nursing 8.4%

Home health 3.5%

Sources: Annual Report of the Board of Trustees of the Federal Supplementary Medical Insurance Trust Fund, 2001; Annual Report of the Board of Trustees of the Federal Hospital Insurance Trust Fund.

FIGURE 8. DEPENDENCY RATIOS (RATIO OF AGE
UNDER 20 AND OVER 65 TO AGE 20–64 POPULATION)

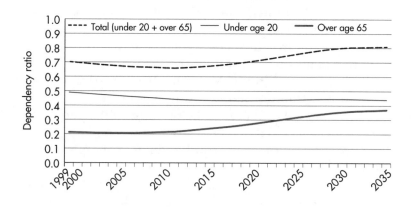

Source: Social Security Administration, Office of the Chief Actuary, available at http://www.ssa.gov/OACT/TR/TR00/lrIndex.html, Table II.H1.

and covered wages. Because Medicare's coverage has not kept pace with the rising medical costs of the elderly, however, an increasing portion of total medical costs has nonetheless been borne by beneficiaries themselves. In Medicare's early years, beneficiaries spent roughly a tenth of their income on out-of-pocket medical costs. By 1999, elderly beneficiaries spent 19 percent of their incomes for health care, while beneficiaries with incomes below the federal poverty line spent fully one-third.[5]

Under current law, moreover, the proportion of Medicare financing borne by beneficiaries will rise. Home health services are being transferred from Part A of Medicare to Part B, and under current law a quarter of these expenditures must be paid for out of enrollee premiums. Independent of this shift, Part B spending is already expected to rise faster than Part A spending, in part because many procedures that once required hospitalization are now done on an outpatient basis. For these reasons, beneficiaries are expected to shoulder an increasing share of spending on services covered by Medicare. The Urban Institute calculates that beneficiary liability for Medicare-related services will rise from 21.4 percent of total program spending in 1998 to more than a quarter of spending in 2025.[6] And these increases do not include the costs of medical items and services not covered by Medicare at all. When these costs are factored in, total out-of-pocket medical spending by elderly Medicare beneficiaries is expected to rise from 18.6 percent of their income in 1998 to 28.6 percent in 2025, assuming that Medicare remains roughly as generous as it is today.[7]

Although Medicare's financial architecture requires adjustment, there are real limits on the share of costs that beneficiaries can be expected to pay. As a group, Medicare beneficiaries are poorly equipped to bear the burden of rising medical expenses. While poverty rates among the elderly are below those of the population as a whole and have declined in recent years, the incomes of Medicare enrollees are clustered in a narrow band above the poverty line.[8] Almost 40 percent of Americans over sixty-five earned less than $16,000 in 1998 (roughly twice the federal poverty level).[9] Moreover, failing to provide adequate protection through Medicare imposes the largest costs on those with the highest medical expenses. Thus, if it were deemed necessary to increase the amount that current beneficiaries pay, it would be preferable to raise the share of program costs financed by beneficiary premiums, which do not vary with medical costs, rather than to reduce the scope of Medicare's protections by limiting coverage or increasing copayments and deductibles.

It must be remembered, too, that most of the medical costs of the elderly and disabled will still have to be met if Medicare does not cover them—whether through the expenditures of beneficiaries and their families, private insurance payments, charity care, the costs to individuals and society of delayed or inadequate care, or other means. If these costs reflect the provision of valuable services whose benefits are judged broadly commensurate with their expense, then the proper question for the nation is not whether those services should be purchased but through what means. Paying for them through Medicare has two advantages over shifting them to other sources. First, although Medicare's cost-control record is hardly unblemished, it has done at least as well as private insurance in containing expenditures while providing inclusive coverage on relatively equal terms to all.[10] It also has a better record of using resources to pay for covered benefits rather than for administrative costs. Second, shifting medical costs for current Medicare enrollees onto alternative sources will almost inevitably place the heaviest burdens on the minority of Medicare beneficiaries with very high medical expenses while posing the greatest financial threat to beneficiaries with lower incomes. These trade-offs can be better understood in the context of some of the specific proposals for restructuring Medicare that have recently been under debate.

MEDICARE REFORM AND MEDICARE FINANCING

The heated debate over Medicare financing has centered primarily on the amount of "savings" different restructuring options might deliver relative to projected future increases in Medicare expenditures. For all the undeniable value of this perspective for considering long-term budgetary effects, it has two significant drawbacks. First, it suggests that there is a reform option that would eliminate Medicare's future financial shortfall without an increase in the revenues devoted to the program. Yet, according to a careful independent analysis conducted by the National Academy of Social Insurance, all Medicare reform plans proposed in recent years, even the most restrictive, "will require additional revenues even after accounting for growth in the overall economy," in part because of the rising proportion of Americans covered by the program.[11]

The second and more serious drawback of focusing only on savings relative to baseline projections is that it tends to bias the debate in favor of one-shot reforms that deliver easily predicted long-term cost reductions and against the sort of incremental cost-saving changes that have been a hallmark of past Medicare revisions.[12] It is a relatively simple task, for example, to forecast long-term savings if Medicare is converted into a "defined contribution" approach in which the amount paid on behalf of beneficiaries is allowed to rise no faster than a predetermined rate. This does not prove, however, that a defined contribution approach will lower the underlying expense of Medicare benefits. If the true cost of benefits grew faster than the defined contribution, savings would only accrue to Medicare if an increasing share of expenditures were borne by beneficiaries themselves. Thus, any assessment of alternative financing arrangements needs to consider not just how they would affect Medicare spending but also how they would allocate the burdens and risks of medical costs more generally.

Although the potential effects are less stark, cost shifting from Medicare to beneficiaries also could very well occur under premium support proposals, such as the 1999 proposal of Senators Breaux and

Frist that was reintroduced in Congress in 2001. This could happen for three primary reasons. First, the level of the government's premium support contribution could be less generous than the current division of Medicare spending and direct beneficiary payments.[13] Second, if the original Medicare program competed alongside private plans, beneficiaries who remained in the original program could well end up paying more for their Medicare coverage than they do now, as would beneficiaries who chose more expensive private health plans. As discussed in the rationale for Principle I, these increases would be particularly troubling if they reflected the segmentation of risk rather than the comparative generosity or efficiency of plans.

Third, a premium support proposal would shift costs to beneficiaries if the amount of the government's contribution failed to keep pace with the rising cost of public or private coverage. Advocates of premium support argue that their approach differs from a pure defined contribution plan in that the level of the government contribution is set through a process of competitive bidding and thus would keep pace with rising premium costs. It is worth noting, however, that the budgetary estimates that have been used to justify the premium support approach assume that private insurance premiums will rise significantly more slowly than Medicare spending— something that has not been true over the past two decades and certainly not over the past few years. It also is worth noting that the premium support approach creates a simple mechanism for reducing the share of Medicare spending that is paid for by the program. Because the proposed reform would move Medicare toward a defined contribution framework in which the federal government paid a set amount toward private or public coverage, it would create a means that does not now exist for potentially shifting Medicare spending onto beneficiaries—namely, allowing the contribution to lag behind the cost of coverage.

While premium support proposals could have the indirect consequence of raising Medicare premiums for some beneficiaries, other reform options seek to make explicit changes in the share of Medicare costs paid by beneficiaries. Perhaps the most prominent of these options is the idea of "means-testing" or "income-scaling" Part B premiums. As noted earlier, all Medicare beneficiaries are already slated to pay a larger share of Medicare expenditures in the future under current law. Some argue, however, that high-income beneficiaries in particular should pay more for their Part B coverage.

   Proposals to scale Part B premiums to income would certainly provide additional revenues for the program. Depending on where the income thresholds were set, several billion dollars annually might be raised.[14] It should be noted, however, that Medicare Part A's financing is already more progressive than Social Security's (because its payroll tax applies to all wages) and that general revenues raised through a progressive income tax are the principal financing source of Medicare Part B. (Part B premiums account for a bit less than 10 percent of Medicare's total revenues.) If Medicare premiums rose for wealthier seniors, moreover, insurers might be able to offer private policies that would induce these often healthier seniors to opt out of the voluntary Part B program. This would shrink the broader Medicare risk pool and possibly jeopardize the political consensus that currently supports the program. Another difficulty is that a premium surcharge for higher-income beneficiaries would have to reach well down the income ladder to raise substantial revenues. According to researchers at the Urban Institute, applying a surcharge to older Americans who earned $50,000 and up would result in just one-third of the revenue that setting the threshold at $30,000—closer to the median income of the elderly—would generate, even though many of the beneficiaries required to pay extra at this lower level would be far from affluent.[15]

   Lowering the projected rate of growth in Medicare spending and increasing the share of program expenditures financed by beneficiaries are two of the three major options for securing the program's long-term finances. The third is increasing the revenues of the program, either by raising taxes or by funding a larger proportion of the program through general revenues. A cornerstone of former President Clinton's 1999 proposal to reform Medicare, for example, was a commitment to transfer roughly $800 billion of the projected budget surplus over the next fifteen years into the program. The administration estimated that this transfer would secure the fiscal health of the Part A trust fund during the years in which the demographic shift caused by the retirement of the baby-boom generation would be the most pronounced.

   Independent of the other changes contained in the Clinton proposal, the commitment to use the surplus to shore up Medicare's fiscal standing is a valuable contribution to the debate for at least two reasons. First, a substantial part of the projected ten-year overall budget surplus of $5.6 trillion is attributable to the slowdown in Medicare and Medicaid spending achieved over the past few years. Second, the argument against using general revenues to improve Medicare's financial standing—that doing so will attenuate the signals needed to encourage fiscal discipline—is weak to the extent that the rising Medicare spending springs from the increasing numbers of beneficiaries. Even very significant reductions in the rate of growth of Medicare spending per capita will not change the reality that the health of the Part A trust fund will decline as a growing share of Americans enroll in the program and fewer workers support it.

As in the past, Medicare's growing costs will need to be addressed through a mix of cost-control efforts, revenue increases, and programmatic reforms. But these growing fiscal needs, reflecting as they do the increasing capacities of medicine and the expanding population that enjoys Medicare's protections, should not be used as justification for radical or ill-considered changes in the program. Because more Americans will be enrolled in Medicare in the coming years, the program will need new revenues. Efforts to keep spending in check should focus first on controlling costs rather than on scaling back benefits. And these efforts should, to the fullest extent possible, not leave older and disabled Americans facing significantly higher medical expenses in the coming decades.

3.

BENEFIT PACKAGE

Principle III. The scope of health care benefits covered under Medicare should be expanded to include elements that are critical to preventing or detecting disease and managing chronic conditions, as well as treating acute illness.

When Medicare was enacted in 1965, its benefits principally covered acute care and were comparable to the coverage offered by private health insurance. Since then, however, the scope of the program's coverage has not kept pace with private insurance, epidemiological developments, or technical advances in health care. Increased longevity and improvements in clinical practice have made the management of chronic illness pivotal. The orientation of the Medicare program and the shape of its benefit package gradually have been adapting to this change, responding to the reality that the provision of health care increasingly takes place outside the hospital. For example, the rules for obtaining home health care through Medicare were liberalized in the late 1980s, while clinical preventive services have been progressively included in the benefit package. Even so, gaps continue to exist between the benefits offered by many private insurance plans and Medicare—a 1997 study estimated that the Medicare package of benefits was less generous than four of five fee-for-service plans offered by large employers.[1]

In light of these developments, outpatient prescription drug coverage—which is a vital part of the treatment of both chronic illnesses and postacute conditions—should be included in the Medicare benefit package. Legislators also should add coverage for additional clinical preventive services that would improve the functioning of seniors and should encourage the Medicare program's efforts to increase the use of existing preventive benefits.

AN OUTPATIENT PRESCRIPTION DRUG BENEFIT

THE GROWING IMPORTANCE OF PRESCRIPTION DRUGS

In the mid-1960s, serious medical conditions were ordinarily treated in a hospital. The affordability of hospital care—not the cost of a cycle of antibiotics or painkillers—was the biggest hurdle facing elderly Americans. The benefit packages of most major insurance plans, such as the Blue Cross and Blue Shield plans on which Medicare was modeled, contained limited coverage of prescription drugs or none at all.

In the past quarter-century, however, outpatient prescription drugs have become central to a wide range of medical therapies (see Figure 9). Their use can prevent the onset or recurrence of major conditions that might otherwise require hospitalization and surgery. For example, beta-blockers have been shown to reduce the risk of heart attacks. Anticoagulants help prevent strokes, especially devastating second

FIGURE 9. ANNUAL PERCENTAGE CHANGE FROM PRIOR YEAR IN SELECTED NATIONAL HEALTH EXPENDITURES

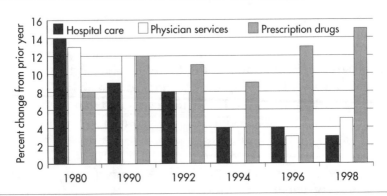

Source: "Prescription Drug Trends," Henry J. Kaiser Family Foundation, Washington, D.C., September 2000, Figure 2.

strokes. Drugs are used to manage chronic conditions and to lower the risk of developing serious complications. Cholesterol-lowering drugs reduce the risk of heart disease, and new medications treat arthritis and osteoporosis more effectively than ever.

Advances in biotechnology are raising hopes for drug therapies that can fight diseases at the genetic level. Such medicines might one day delay the onset of Alzheimer's disease, which currently affects 4 million older Americans, a number that could grow to 14.3 million in the year 2050 if no advances in its treatment occur.[2]

Prescription drugs are especially important to older Americans. Largely because they suffer from treatable chronic illnesses like diabetes, hypertension, and arthritis at a much higher rate than younger Americans, seniors use more prescription drugs than any other age group. They account for about a third of all purchases of medicines, taking an average of twenty-one prescriptions annually. Seniors with insurance coverage use more than twenty-two prescriptions a year, while those without coverage take an average of seventeen prescriptions.[3] As with all medical services, intensive users account for the bulk of prescription drug use—7 percent of beneficiaries account for 32 percent of all beneficiary spending,[4] and three-quarters of this spending goes toward roughly one-third of beneficiaries.[5] However, about nine of every ten younger beneficiaries, those aged sixty-five to seventy, also report taking at least one prescription drug on a regular basis.[6]

WHAT COVERAGE CURRENTLY EXISTS FOR PEOPLE ON MEDICARE? WHY DOES IT MATTER?

In 1998, about 73 percent of Medicare beneficiaries had drug coverage for at least some of the year (see Figure 10, page 50).[7] A substantial number of beneficiaries lack stable drug coverage, possibly reflecting changes in private insurance markets and the tendency for some beneficiaries to purchase coverage only when they expect to need it most. Using 1996 data, one group of researchers estimated that slightly fewer than 53 percent of beneficiaries had continuous coverage.[8] Lower-income Medicare beneficiaries are less able or likely to purchase insurance that includes coverage for prescription drugs than those with higher incomes: three of five beneficiaries with incomes above 250 percent of the poverty line report

FIGURE 10. SOURCES OF PRESCRIPTION DRUG COVERAGE FOR MEDICARE BENEFICIARIES, 1998

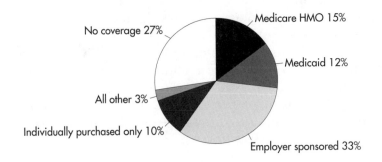

Note: Data are limited to Medicare beneficiaries living in the community.
Source: John A. Poisal and Lauren Murray, "Growing Differences between Medicare Beneficiaries with and without Drug Coverage," *Health Affairs* 20, no. 2 (March/April 2001): 74–85.

having insurance that included a drug benefit; just two of five below this line make the same claim.[9]

Medicare beneficiaries are the only major insured group in the United States that lack drug coverage through their primary insurer. Among the U.S. population under sixty-five, 77 percent had drug coverage, mostly through their employer or the Medicaid program.[10] Most of the adults under age sixty-five who lack prescription drug coverage are without health insurance altogether.

Why does being uninsured for outpatient drug coverage matter? It matters because uninsured seniors and disabled Americans pay much more for drugs than their insured counterparts and may lack access to medications that can improve their health. Seniors as a group pay for fully half of their drug spending out-of-pocket, compared to 34 percent for the under-sixty-five population.[11] Among beneficiaries, those without insurance coverage paid an average of $546 out-of-pocket in 1998, compared with $325 for the insured.[12] The uninsured spend less on prescriptions overall but pay a larger amount out-of-pocket (see Figure 11). A small percentage of beneficiaries face very high drug expenditures: roughly 10 percent of beneficiaries are expected to incur in excess of $4000 in annual prescription drug expenditures in 2001.[13] The uninsured also pay

FIGURE 11. OUT-OF-POCKET AND INSURER SPENDING ON PRESCRIPTION DRUGS BY MEDICARE BENEFICIARIES BY TYPE OF DRUG COVERAGE, 1996

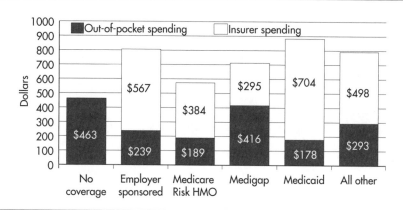

Sources: Information and Methods Group, Office of Strategic Planning, Health Care Financing Administration; Health Care Financing Administration, *Medicare Current Beneficiary Survey,* Cost and Use File, 1996.

higher prices for their drugs than the insured since managed care plans and employers are generally able to negotiate discounts based on the volume of purchases made on behalf of their policyholders.[14]

Lack of coverage and high cost sharing for prescription drugs can result in Medicare beneficiaries consuming fewer medically necessary drugs.[15] For example, a recent study of Medicare enrollees suffering from hypertension, which if untreated can greatly increase the risk of strokes, heart disease, and kidney failure, found that those without drug coverage were 40 percent more likely not to purchase any antihypertensive medicines than those with drug coverage.[16] Disparities in the number of prescriptions taken are much greater between lower-income beneficiaries who have drug coverage and those who lack such coverage compared to their higher-income counterparts.[17] A study that examined the results of adding a prescription drug benefit to the health care program of the Canadian province of Ontario found that drug use increased most for poorer beneficiaries, who generally have the greatest health care needs.[18]

Studies conducted by the PRIME Institute at the University of Minnesota for Families USA, a consumer advocacy organization, conclude that prices for the fifty prescription drugs most commonly used by seniors have risen markedly over the past decade and in the past year. The authors estimate that the price of prescription drugs most frequently used by older Americans rose 30.5 percent on average from January 1994 to January 2000, nearly double the 15.4 percent inflation rate, and that six of the thirty-nine most popular drugs that were on the market during this entire time period increased in price five times faster than inflation (see Figure 12 for growth in the price of prescription drugs used by all Americans).[19] Since many seniors live on fixed incomes that rise based on the consumer price index, these increases suggest that the rising cost of prescription drugs has crowded out other spending, such as buying food or other essentials.

As the clinical uses for drugs are increasing, the current sources of supplemental insurance coverage for drugs, such as employer-sponsored retiree programs, Medigap plans, and Medicare HMO plans, are becoming increasingly more costly, less generous, and less available. (The background paper by Thomas Rice takes up this issue in more detail.) Within Medicare+Choice, 68 percent of plans provided some drug coverage in 2000, down from 73 percent a year earlier. The number of plans charging a premium jumped from 42

FIGURE 12. GROWTH IN PRESCRIPTION DRUG PRICES COMPARED TO GENERAL INFLATION

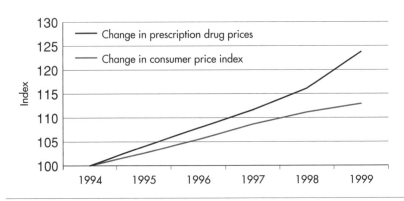

Source: "An Outpatient Prescription Drug Benefit for Medicare," Idea Brief no. 10, The Century Foundation, New York, June 2000.

percent to 62 percent in the same time period, much of this owing to
the increased rate and cost of pharmaceutical use.[20] Moreover, withdrawals of Medicare+Choice plans from various markets, which
began in 1998, have continued through 2001, making drug coverage through this option increasingly less available or affordable.[21] In
2001, service withdrawals affecting 934,000 beneficiaries were
expected to occur, with about 159,000 of these people on Medicare
left without an HMO option in their area. Plans that remain in the
program are tending to increase premiums and reduce benefit caps.
The 2000 terminations affected poorer beneficiaries the most: 73
percent of those whose plans no longer contract with Medicare had
incomes of $20,000 or less, and 38 percent had less than a high
school education, a much lower proportion compared with the profile of Medicare+Choice beneficiaries as a group.[22]

Employer-sponsored drug coverage is usually the most generous, and more beneficiaries obtain supplemental drug coverage through their former employers than through any other form
of insurance. But the number of large companies offering retiree
benefits fell from 80 percent to 66 percent from 1991 to 1999,
with other companies considering dropping or sharply reducing
coverage.[23] The rise in company spending on prescription drugs
has been one of the biggest concerns prompting the scaling down
of employer-sponsored retiree coverage; this trend appears to be
continuing.

Fewer than 10 percent of Medicare beneficiaries now purchase
supplemental Medigap polices that include some drug coverage
along with other protections against Medicare cost sharing and benefit gaps. Just three of the ten tightly regulated plans (known as
plans A through J) include a drug benefit—which requires a
deductible and is capped at 50 percent of spending up to $2500
under the most generous plan. Adverse selection has resulted in
extremely high premiums for the dwindling number of seniors who
elect to buy these policies. Medigap rates range considerably by state
and age of beneficiary. Comparing plans F and J (which are similar
except for the inclusion of $3000 of drug coverage in the latter) in
all states, however, shows the very large effects of drug coverage on
premiums across the board. For example, a sixty-five-year-old
Connecticut resident would pay $1426 for Plan F, compared to $2924
for Plan J. Medigap increasingly resembles prepayment for drugs
rather than genuine insurance.[24]

PRICE, UTILIZATION, AND COST OF PRESCRIPTION DRUGS

While drugs are more essential to the well-being of the elderly than ever before, they are becoming more expensive and less affordable for seniors. In considerable part, this reflects strong demand for new drugs among both elderly and nonelderly Americans. Consumers and physicians often desire these new pharmaceutical products because they are more effective and have fewer side effects than the drugs they replace. (Some evidence suggests that the elderly are more likely to suffer side effects and to fail to benefit from switching among medicines that have similar therapeutic benefits for young people.[25]) Partly as a result of Food and Drug Administration rulings and other regulatory changes, more new drugs have been approved and have entered the market in the past few years than ever before.[26] Demand for these new products is stimulated through aggressive direct marketing to consumers—on television and in print ads—and high-powered salesmanship aimed at doctors and managed care plans. Pharmaceutical companies spent an estimated $1.3 billion on direct marketing and $7 billion to market drugs to physicians in 1998.

Increased spending on prescription drugs has arisen from the substitution of higher-priced new drugs for older ones, inflation in the prices of both newer and older drugs, and higher overall utilization of prescriptions concentrated on the newer products. According to a report released by the National Institute of Health Care Management (NIHCM), "In 1998, the average price per prescription for new drugs was $71.49, more than twice the average $30.47 price for previously existing drugs." This NIHCM study attributed 42 percent of the spending increases between 1992 and 1998 to the introduction of expensive new drugs, 22 percent to price rises for older drugs, and 36 percent to increased use of these drugs (see Figure 13).[27]

In some cases, the availability of prescription drug coverage might save money for the health care system as a whole. Spending on drugs that substitute directly for acute care, such as treating ulcers with medication rather than surgery, is one way this can happen. On a per episode basis, acute care is usually more expensive than drug therapies. One economist has estimated that an increase of one hundred prescriptions might be correlated with 16.3 fewer patient days spent in the hospital, with potential savings from a greater use of drug therapy partially offset by a spending increase on ambulatory care.[28]

FIGURE 13. PERCENTAGE CONTRIBUTION OF CHANGES IN PRICE AND UTILIZATION TO INCREASE IN PRESCRIPTION DRUG SPENDING, 1993–98

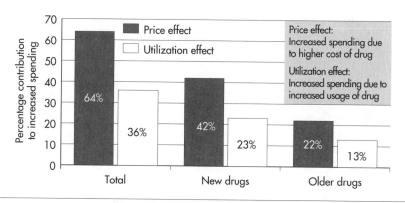

Source: "Factors Affecting the Growth of Prescription Drug Expenditures," report prepared by Barents Group LLC for the National Institute for Health Care Management Research and Educational Foundation, Washington, D.C., July 9, 1999, p. v, Table B.

Depending on the particular drug and the condition of patients, the availability of prescription drugs can sometimes prevent chronically ill patients from needing institutionalization, which is often more costly and lowers the quality of life for older Americans. When the state of New Hampshire cut drug payments in its Medicaid program, for example, a follow-up study found that the chronically ill elderly who were affected by these cuts were twice as likely as a control group to enter nursing homes.[29] The cuts in drug spending on this group ultimately cost the state more than it saved.

While the introduction of an outpatient prescription drug benefit will probably reduce Medicare's spending on some other medical services, overall Medicare spending will increase after a drug benefit is enacted.[30] Since the utilization of services usually increases with insurance coverage, spending on the drug benefit also is likely to increase over time, especially if newer drugs are routinely covered. Spending on pharmaceuticals, which has risen rapidly for private insurers, is largely responsible for the recent rise in the premiums they charge and for an increase in overall health care spending.[31]

Studies that assess the cost-effectiveness of different medications may be useful in helping to justify higher spending and in distinguishing between drugs that have a greater or lesser impact on the health of seniors. While the effects of treatments on health outcomes are difficult to measure precisely—and quality-of-life measures are among the most elusive—such studies can be helpful in assessing the marginal benefit of medications for seniors and the disabled. For example, one study suggested that the drug warfarin, when prescribed in lieu of aspirin for patients with certain kinds of risk factors for stroke, resulted in a much lower ratio of spending per "quality-adjusted life year"(QALY) gained for patients over seventy-five than for those over sixty-five.[32] One survey of the literature on cost-effectiveness research on drugs has found that 11 percent of the medications being researched actually saved money for a particular health care program, while other medications provided important benefits for moderate extra costs.[33]

Most plans for a Medicare drug benefit try to include incentives that encourage the cost-conscious use of clinically appropriate drugs and discourage wasteful or dangerous use of medications. Different versions of these strategies are carried out by pharmacy benefit managers in the U.S. private sector or are employed by health care systems elsewhere in the world. While many questions about how these strategies could be adapted to Medicare remain, some of the most promising and important approaches include:[34]

- Managing a formulary, or a list of drugs that are approved by a particular insurer. Some restrictive formularies limit coverage to only those drugs on the list. Others require higher co-payments for certain brand-name drugs. A tiered system, in which beneficiaries pay a fixed copayment or a percentage of the price for more expensive drugs in a particular category, is becoming more common. National health programs in some countries peg their reimbursements to the cost of a particular preferred medication in a therapeutic category, a practice known as "reference pricing."

- Encouraging the use of generic drugs, chemical compounds that have the same composition as brand-name drugs but are no longer under patent protection. Generics are generally less expensive than innovator drugs. Studies have found that if multiple generic drugs in a category come onto the market to compete with a brand-name drug, the price of the latter will fall.[35] Many brand-name drugs will be coming off patent in the next decade. However, manufacturers of generics lack market clout. Moreover, pharmaceutical companies usually promote their newest and most lucrative drugs even when they sell a generic version as well.[36]

- Developing and installing information systems for pharmacists to help prevent adverse interactions between different drugs prescribed for seniors and to curb redundant use. Medicare might choose to screen out inappropriate use by paying for medication reviews by pharmacists, which it does not do at present.[37] The program also could help prevent misuse of drugs by providing more information about proper medication management directly to beneficiaries.

DESIGNING A MEDICARE PRESCRIPTION DRUG BENEFIT

Designing and enacting a Medicare drug benefit will be a delicate balancing act. The aim for policymakers will be ensuring that Medicare beneficiaries can afford medically necessary drugs while limiting the burden of additional costs to taxpayers. The possible effects of a benefit on pharmaceutical company revenues need to be carefully weighed as well. Some of these revenues are used to finance the research and development of promising new drugs, and the likelihood of a strong return on investment attracts new capital investment for innovation.

Different designs for a drug benefit try to balance these goals in different ways. This reflects their backers' assessment of the costs of new programs, their effect on existing coverage, and the impact on the pharmaceutical industry—as well as broader philosophical considerations about the appropriate scope of government.[38] The most important distinction between these designs is whether they offer a universal benefit or attempt to target the benefit toward lower-income beneficiaries. Some designs that figure prominently in recent or current legislation involve:

- subsidies to state pharmaceutical assistance programs for low-income beneficiaries;

- subsidies given to existing insurers through the private market-place;[39]

- a restructured Medicare program in which competing plans offer drug benefits; and

- a universal benefit within Medicare, perhaps similar to the existing Part B program for physicians' and outpatient services.

Since a large and growing literature compares these approaches and tries to model the effects on prices, utilization, access, and overall cost of the particular plans based on them, this report will limit itself to summarizing these designs' main advantages and disadvantages.[40]

The principal advantage of subsidizing existing state pharmaceutical assistance programs (which presently operate in sixteen states and are planned in six more) is that the programs will be less expensive than more comprehensive reforms and may target the most needy. The drawback is that programs would have to be developed from scratch in many states; some qualifying individuals would not get assistance because they would not apply for benefits, and a number of less well-off Medicare beneficiaries with demonstrable need probably would not qualify under eligibility guidelines. Moreover, existing pharmacy benefit programs have funding caps that limit the number of eligible beneficiaries who can actually get help.

Subsidizing existing insurers shares the virtues of using a structure that is already in place to deliver benefits and the promise of giving more immediate aid. The problems of this approach mirror the adverse selection problems that have plagued Medigap plans: sicker beneficiaries would presumably seek out insurers that offer drug coverage, driving up costs and premiums. Anticipating this result, insurers have publicly expressed reservations about offering freestanding drug coverage for seniors.[41]

The third strategy relies fundamentally on a major overhaul of the Medicare program to increase competition among private health plans. The premium support legislation first introduced by Senators Breaux and Frist in the 106th Congress (S. 1895) and reintroduced in the 107th Congress (S.357) is one such plan. It requires plans to offer drug coverage in "high-option" plans, each with its own premium. Since this reform proposal would involve such major across-the-board changes to Medicare, its specific potential impact on drug coverage is hard to assess. The promise is that competition among plans would result in lower and attractive premiums for beneficiaries. The risk is that premiums would rise rapidly for high-option plans, making them less affordable, and that mechanisms for relieving the burden on lower-income Medicare recipients would prove inadequate.

The main advantages of a universal benefit are that it would result in the broadest access to drug insurance for seniors, pool risk among the most recipients, and carry on Medicare's tradition of offering a single benefit package to all those eligible. The benefit's principal drawback is its potential overall cost. A universal benefit could accelerate the decline in employer-sponsored coverage, as companies try to shift costs to the public payer, resulting in even higher expenditures than projected.

The proposal by former President Clinton calls for a voluntary drug benefit within Medicare that would resemble the existing Part B program. Proponents of a voluntary benefit believe that premiums could be set low enough, and subsidies made generous enough, that this benefit would attract near-universal enrollment. However, no voluntary benefit can escape the potential problem of adverse selection altogether. A mandatory drug benefit (such as through making participation in Medicare conditional on accepting the benefit and its method of financing) would solve the adverse selection problem but would face opposition from those satisfied with their current sources of coverage.

All these designs for a drug benefit, including those for offering targeted low-income coverage, would represent an improvement over the status quo. A universal benefit, however, would be the most compatible with the social insurance design of Medicare and the program's history of offering a common benefit package to all eligible recipients. Targeting low-income beneficiaries faces several additional problems.[42] Subsidies to programs for the poor and near-poor, in particular the Qualified Medicare Beneficiary (QMB) and Specified Low-Income Medicare Beneficiary (SLMB) programs, have not attracted a high percentage of eligible recipients. A drug benefit covered within Medicare would likely have a much higher enrollment rate. Moreover, wealth and income are more evenly distributed among the elderly than in other age groups. Since no single group of "poor" elderly stands out from the rest, eligibility cutoff lines would be fairly arbitrary, perhaps promoting "gaming" in order to qualify.

Any of these benefit designs, including a limit on out-of-pocket expenses, would help restore the program's founding purpose of protection against the potentially ruinous costs of health care.[43] This feature would be especially desirable for assisting the 10 percent of beneficiaries who spend more than $4000 annually on prescription drugs.[44]

PREVENTIVE SERVICES

Preventing the decline or loss of basic functions among seniors — such as the ability to feed or dress oneself—is a critical aim of geriatric care. It is especially important for patients with multiple chronic illnesses.[45] Covering outpatient prescription drugs through Medicare would help move the program in the direction of promoting better health among the elderly and disabled rather than principally insuring against the costs of medical care. Adding certain preventive services to the Medicare benefit package and encouraging the use of existing services also would promote this aim.

Because Medicare was originally designed around standard insurance principles that emphasize indemnifying against major and unexpected events rather than paying for routine and predictable health needs, the coverage of preventive services by the program is a relatively recent development.[46] The first preventive service, pneumococcal pneumonia vaccine, was added to the benefit package in 1980. Better prevention may save money for Medicare in the long run if the disability rate of older beneficiaries continues to decline, but maintaining healthy functioning for the elderly would be the principal aim of improved preventive benefits.[47]

Preventive and early-detection services still tend to be underused by people on Medicare. Many older Americans, for example, miss out on routine tests for colon cancer. In 1992, only 30 percent of people fifty years of age and over reported having received a fecal occult blood test within the preceding two years.[48] The U.S. Preventive Services Task Force recommends that this test be administered on an annual basis to people over the age of sixty-five. Data developed by HCFA indicate that only fifty-six white and forty-nine black enrollees out of every one thousand received a colonoscopy, a more powerful diagnostic test for this cancer, in 1996.[49] Proper screenings for this second-leading cancer killer in the United States could reduce fatalities. The frequency of vaccinations and early-warning diagnostic tests for Medicare beneficiaries also falls beneath desirable rates across the board.[50]

The Balanced Budget Act of 1997 did add a number of prevention initiatives to Medicare, such as annual mammography screening, prostate and colorectal cancer screening, and bone mass measurements.[51] This act also reduced many of the coinsurance and deductible payment requirements on these preventive services, though some copayments remain.[52] Legislation pending at the time of writing would widen coverage of mammographies, as well as expand coverage of colonoscopies and cover eye examinations to detect glaucoma.[53] The Institute of Medicine has recommended that Medicare cover outpatient nutrition therapy and broaden the definition of "medically necessary" dental services.[54] Better Medicare coverage of services related to sensory impairment also could improve the functioning and social participation of many seniors.[55]

Beyond adding new preventive benefits that meet standards of clinical effectiveness and fiscal prudence, the government should embark on a campaign to educate Medicare beneficiaries about what is now covered in this area and about the potential importance of using these benefits.

Revamping Medicare's benefit package will not be inexpensive. It seems reasonable, however, that elderly and disabled Americans should have access to comprehensive health coverage that is comparable to that offered to many working-age Americans. Covering preventive services could make the difference between autonomy and dependence for many seniors. Medications can permit patients to return to normal routines after being hospitalized and can improve their quality of life. Including drug coverage will help preserve Medicare's original purpose of protecting against the high costs of essential medical care while possibly helping reduce other medical costs and improving the functioning of older Americans.

4.

VULNERABLE POPULATIONS

Principle IV. Proposals to reform Medicare should reduce and eliminate, rather than maintain or exacerbate, the disadvantages faced by vulnerable populations within the program.

Medicare was designed to improve access to medical care among the elderly and the disabled. Relative to the difficulties in receiving care that many seniors faced prior to its existence, it has succeeded admirably. Since Medicare was enacted, gaps in hospital admissions and in medical services received have narrowed dramatically between the elderly and nonelderly and among different subgroups of older Americans.[1]

Nonetheless, various groups of Americans eligible for Medicare still face disparities in their access to care and in the quality of treatment they receive.[2] These groups, which overlap substantially, include:

- racial and ethnic minorities, notably African-Americans and Hispanics;

- low-income beneficiaries, such as "dual eligibles" who qualify for Medicare and Medicaid;

- older and frailer beneficiaries, especially older women, who are at risk for disabilities stemming from chronic illness; and[3]

- rural populations.

Given Medicare's universal character as a social insurance program that supports access to good quality care for all its beneficiaries, maintaining and improving services for these "vulnerable populations" should be a subject of considerable concern. Because individuals with these characteristics tend to be poorer and in worse health than the average Medicare beneficiary, reforms to the program that might increase the amount that they pay out-of-pocket for health care or that might impose other barriers to access would hurt them disproportionately. For this reason, reforms that could jeopardize access to care and worsen existing disadvantages should not be pursued unless strong protections against their negative potential consequences can be fashioned. On the other hand, additions to the benefit package and changes to reimbursement policies that improve access to providers may help vulnerable groups more than other people in Medicare.

RACIAL AND ETHNIC MINORITIES

Since the availability of health insurance is probably the single most important factor in equalizing access to care, it is not surprising that health differences by race and ethnicity within Medicare pale in comparison to those observed in the working-age population.[4] Nevertheless, despite formal equality of coverage, disparities in health status and health outcomes between whites and African-Americans and Hispanics eligible for Medicare remain.

For example, researchers report that African-American beneficiaries are receiving fewer Medicare services than they are estimated to need in several clinical areas, such as certain elective procedures for treating heart disease and kidney failure. The rate at which preventive services are used, including screening for breast and colon cancer, also is significantly lower for black Medicare recipients (see Figure 14).[5]

Hispanics eligible for Medicare are nearly twice as likely to rate their health status as fair or poor as older whites. Moreover, the income of nearly one in three Hispanic beneficiaries was below the poverty line in 1996, compared to that of about one in ten white Medicare recipients. Latino beneficiaries also were more likely to suffer from cognitive impairments and disabilities and less likely to use many preventive services than whites.[6]

Older Americans who belong to a racial or ethnic minority are less likely to purchase supplemental insurance than white Medicare

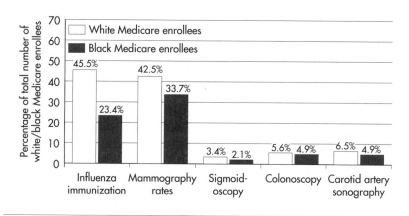

FIGURE 14. PREVENTIVE AND DIAGNOSTIC SERVICE RATES FOR MEDICARE ENROLLEES AGE 65 AND OVER, BY RACE, 1996

Source: Marian E. Gornick, *Vulnerable Populations and Medicare Services: Why Do Disparities Exist?* (New York: The Century Foundation Press, 2000), Tables 4.2–4.4.

beneficiaries or to receive employer-sponsored retiree coverage.[7] Older minority individuals are almost twice as likely as whites to rely on Medicare alone for their health insurance coverage.[8]

The poorer health of racial and ethnic minorities on Medicare clearly reflects in large part their prior relationship to the U.S. health care system. Minority Americans under the age of sixty-five are much less likely than whites to have health insurance: 31 percent lack insurance, as opposed to 14 percent of whites.[9] They are more likely to suffer from disabilities and chronic illness and to die sooner. Black men, for example, are 40 percent more likely to have heart disease than white men, and they experience stroke at nearly twice the rate of whites.[10] Though many of these differences narrow when socioeconomic differences are controlled for, they persist at each level of income.[11]

Raising the eligibility age for Medicare would be especially hard on racial and ethnic minorities. They are more likely to have worked in manual occupations or in lower-paying service sector jobs; in some cases, they never had access to steady health insurance coverage until Medicare became available to them. Because they have lower incomes and fewer resources on average than whites and are more likely to be in poor health, they are consequently less likely to be able to purchase affordable individual insurance policies as they approach retirement age. While

49 percent of white workers above the age of sixty, for example, reported being in very good or excellent health, just 29 percent of black workers said the same.[12]

Low-Income Medicare Beneficiaries

Some Medicare beneficiaries with incomes below the poverty line qualify for full Medicaid coverage; others with incomes just above this level may have their Part B premiums and cost sharing paid for in full or part by state Medicaid programs.

Especially for these "dual eligibles" with full Medicaid coverage, such assistance can sharply reduce the out-of-pocket health spending burdens associated with paying for Medicare. One study estimates that such out-of-pocket spending averaged just 4 percent of annual income for those in this category. For those just above the poverty line (100–125 percent of poverty), the comparable figure for out-of-

Figure 15. Average Out-of-Pocket Spending on Health Care by Medicare Beneficiaries Age 65 and Older as Percentage of Income, 1999 Projections

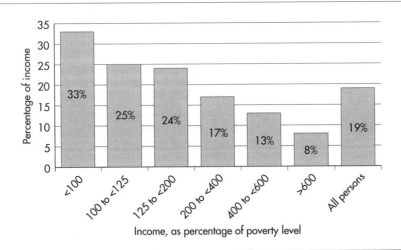

Source: U.S. Congress, House, Committee on Ways and Means, 2000 Green Book (Washington, D.C.: U.S. Government Printing Office, 2000), Appendix B, Table B-12.

FIGURE 16. CHRONIC CONDITIONS OF ELDERLY PERSONS BY FAMILY INCOME, 1995

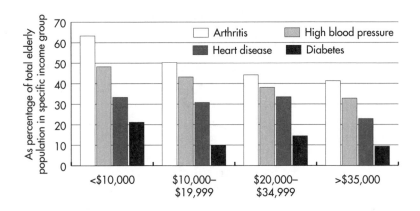

Source: U.S. Congress, House, Committee on Ways and Means, *2000 Green Book* (Washington, D.C.: U.S. Government Printing Office, 2000), Appendix B, Table B-3.

pocket health spending was 23 percent of income.[13] To be sure, beneficiaries in this income range are eligible for partial assistance through Medicaid, but many fail to apply for such assistance. The consumer advocacy group Families USA estimates, for instance, that as many as 3.9 million Americans who may be eligible for such assistance have failed to obtain it.[14]

This suggests that new strategies—and possibly more federal funding—for outreach should be considered in order to encourage enrollment of the many low-income Medicare beneficiaries who are currently eligible for but not participating in these state-assistance programs.

The income distribution of Medicare beneficiaries shows that the income of many elderly and disabled Americans falls into a range just above the level at which they are eligible for assistance. For these Americans, increases in Medicare copayments and premiums and out-of-pocket spending are especially burdensome (see Figures 15 and 16). They also are hardest hit by changes in the availability of supplemental coverage through former employers or Medicare managed care plans.

Premium support proposals would offer beneficiaries a fixed payment from the government that they would use toward paying the premium of competing health plans. Should health plans with modest premiums and expanded benefit packages become more widely available in the future, these plans might help those low-income beneficiaries who do not qualify for assistance with cost sharing and premium payments. Beneficiaries with modest incomes appear to have enrolled at a higher rate than average in existing Medicare+Choice plans, presumably in large measure to obtain additional benefits at a low extra cost.[15] However, as noted in Chapter 1, implementation of premium support proposals could undermine the universal character of Medicare and could hurt some low-income individuals the most. This might happen if sicker patients clustered in the fee-for-service program, confronting higher premiums and out-of-pocket costs, a situation that could occur as a result of adverse selection and ineffective risk-adjustment procedures. This outcome would be the most problematic for older Medicare beneficiaries and patients with chronic illnesses, who have been the most likely to remain enrolled in fee-for-service Medicare to date.

OLDER, FRAILER, AND DISABLED RECIPIENTS

As beneficiaries age, spending on medical care tends to account for a larger share of their income. Medicare beneficiaries over the age of eighty-five are most likely to rely exclusively on Medicare. They more often lack employer-sponsored supplemental insurance or individually purchased supplemental insurance. They also use more home health and nursing services and have a greater need for long-term care (which is not covered by Medicare). Older beneficiaries are more likely to suffer from chronic and disabling conditions such as arthritis and hypertension, as well as functional impairments such as incontinence.

Women are especially at risk. They account for more than 70 percent of the over-eighty-five population, reflecting the fact that women's life expectancy in the United States is almost seven years longer than men's at birth and three years longer at age sixty-five. Older women suffer from poorer health and are worse off financially than older men: about two-thirds of Medicare beneficiaries with functional impairments are women. Women over the age of eighty-five spend 27 percent of their income out-of-pocket on health care, compared to 17 percent for the average person on Medicare.[16] Researchers from the Urban Institute estimate that older women in poor health, who currently spend more than half of their income on health care, will spend 72 percent of their income on health care by 2025 if current trends in medical spending and Medicare policy continue.[17]

Enhancing the benefit package would reduce hardship for some low-income, minority, and older Medicare beneficiaries. For instance, Americans over the age of sixty-five with incomes of less than $15,000 spent 16.6 percent of their incomes on out-of-pocket outpatient prescription drugs in 1998.[18] As Chapter 3 explored in more detail, most comprehensive drug benefit proposals under consideration in the 106th Congress, including the Clinton and Breaux-Frist plans, featured a sliding scale for premiums that would assist these lower-income citizens. Modernizing the benefit package also should reduce the demand and need for individually purchased supplemental insurance. As the background paper by Thomas Rice in this volume shows, such coverage is becoming progressively more expensive and harder to obtain, features that affect low-income and minority beneficiaries most adversely.

Placing a limit on out-of-pocket spending, a provision resembling the "stop-loss" provisions found in most private insurance plans, would be especially advantageous for older and sicker beneficiaries. Such beneficiaries, on average, are more likely to fall ill and to have lower incomes. Consequently, they are more likely to incur larger out-of-pocket Medicare expenses—especially through cost sharing for hospital stays or prescription drug purchases—and to have trouble paying their bills.[19]

Redesigning the program's current reimbursement and coverage policies so that they better encourage the coordination of care and the continuity of care (defined as providing the optimal mix of services at a given time and over time and encouraging a stable relationship with one or more particular providers[20]) also could be of great benefit to older Americans with chronic illnesses and functional disabilities.[21]

Because Medicare was designed principally to pay for acute care delivered in a hospital, its benefit package is not well suited for seniors who suffer from multiple chronic illnesses that may best be treated through frequent, low-tech interventions and monitoring rather than through hospitalization or surgery.[22] Though preventing complications and functional decline brought on by chronic illness is one of the most important goals in caring for Medicare enrollees, the Medicare benefit package does not cover most routine physical exams or vision, dental, or hearing exams, even though the degradation of these faculties is closely associated with depression, the loss of motor skills, and more serious conditions.[23]

Medicare rules aimed at preventing overbilling and fraud—an important goal—may, however, have the inadvertent consequence of hindering the optimal treatment of Medicare-eligible patients who need both nursing home care and acute care.[24] As Gail Warden, the president of the Henry Ford Health System, observes, "Nursing home residents who experience an acute event, such as one requiring antibiotic treatments for an infection, must be hospitalized for three days before the nursing home can provide them with skilled care, in the same facility."[25] The frail patient must move between facilities—facing potential threats to health such as infections in the hospital—and must deal with multiple providers. Likewise, task force member Dr. Al Siu of the Mount Sinai School of Medicine described a situation in which Medicare's home health payment policies are an obstacle to providing care that acknowledges the patient's medical and social needs:

> We thought it would be a good idea for the doctors to actually be there at the same time as the visiting nurses on that first day when the patient goes home. The problem is that Medicare wouldn't allow us to bill both services if they were there at the same time, or even on the same day. If the patient had been dragged to the office and a visiting nurse happened to be there on the same day, Medicare would allow that to be billed as two separate bills. But Medicare would not allow us to have both visits paid for when they are on the same day, let alone at the same time. It's an example of how the package and the rules will drive care.

The quality of care given to older and frailer Medicare beneficiaries also could be improved through a higher level of federal funding for geriatric research and the expansion of fellowship programs for physicians who specialize in aging. Just nine thousand geriatric specialists are currently certified in the United States and only $100 million of the National Institutes of Health's roughly $15 billion budget goes to the broader study of aging.[26]

Chapter 6 explores in more detail the development and refinement of outreach efforts aimed at beneficiaries and the provision of information to them about Medicare's benefits and coverage policies. Developing effective and culturally sensitive material is likely to be critical for the most vulnerable beneficiaries, who often have received less formal education and suffer from more cognitive difficulties than the average beneficiary.[27] For example, because almost half of women over the age of eighty-five who remain in the community live alone, they are likely to have limited assistance when making decisions about their health insurance coverage. Competition-based reforms that rely heavily on consumers to distinguish between the value of their health options should focus on the extent to which the need for information and the capacity to process it differs among people on Medicare.

RURAL POPULATIONS

Medicare's efforts to ensure access to high-quality care frequently run into difficulties in the process of serving rural beneficiaries.[28] The most important reason is the variation in the supply of hospitals and doctors. Fewer doctors, especially specialists, practice in rural areas, and single community hospitals frequently serve large regions. States with the highest per capita Medicare spending (such as New York, Florida, California, and Texas) are more urbanized; those with lower spending (such as Idaho, New Mexico, Iowa, Maine, and Vermont) are generally rural.[29] To be sure, much of the additional spending reflects varying physician practice styles and the overall health of a state's population, but it also reflects the fact that urban residents can and do get more medical services.

In addition, Medicare managed care plans have been slow to move into rural areas, largely because their payments have reflected lower fee-for-service prices and because it is hard to build provider networks in these areas. In 1998, just five "high-payment" urban states accounted for 57 percent of Medicare managed care enrollment, while the six states that lacked a single Medicare managed care plan were predominantly rural (Alaska, Mississippi, Montana, South Dakota, Vermont, and Wyoming).[30] Beneficiaries in these states have not received the additional benefits at little additional cost that residents of states with higher payment rates have enjoyed.[31]

The disadvantages faced by rural Medicare beneficiaries—both under the existing system and under reforms based on plan choice and competition—stem principally from the relatively small number of doctors who practice in rural America and the tradition of relatively lower costs in these areas. Operating in rural areas has not proved attractive for health plans, largely because putting together a provider network is difficult and because reimbursements, based on fee-for-service Medicare payments, have historically been low.[32] These circumstances relating to rural beneficiaries could pose special problems for structural reforms to the program that emphasize provider competition and plan choice. Fewer providers mean fewer opportunities for plans to construct competing networks and to capture the efficiencies and lower prices (and program savings) that could result. Fewer patient visits mean that rural providers have little incentive or opportunity to lower their fees in return for the promise of higher patient volume that managed care networks characteristically promise. Since rural populations depend to an even greater degree on traditional Medicare than beneficiaries who live in urban and suburban areas, any premium increases associated with adverse selection will affect them disproportionately.

To the extent that discrepancies in access to providers for older and disabled Americans living in rural areas reflect the career choices of medical professionals, there is little that Medicare can do directly to redress them. Congress and program administrators have attempted to narrow the gaps between Medicare managed care payment rates in urban and rural counties by calculating them based on a "blend" of national and local rates, a process initiated by the Balanced Budget Act of 1997. Subsequent legislation has raised the "floor" payment to plans in rural areas and has offered modest bonus payments to plans that choose to enter a county in which no other Medicare+Choice plan is currently operating. To date, these measures have not achieved their intended result of attracting Medicare HMOs to rural areas.[33] Since rural beneficiaries, unlike some of their urban counterparts, have not been able to obtain additional benefits at little or no extra cost, they will be especially helped by any improvements to the comprehensiveness of the basic benefit package. Moreover, the program could do several things to help rectify possible imbalances in access and quality of care for rural beneficiaries.[34] It should closely monitor the prospective payments received by rural hospitals, which have lower overall margins on average than urban hospitals. And it should step up its efforts to disseminate guidelines for best medical practices in the hope that these standards can help equalize the quality of medical treatment nationwide.

CONCLUSION

Since all older and disabled Americans share a common vulnerability to the effects of aging and its associated risk of higher medical costs, the impact of reforms on different beneficiaries may differ more in degree than in kind. However, the most vulnerable people on Medicare depend more heavily than the norm on the protections that Medicare offers. Their lower incomes and poorer health status, on the whole, put them at greater risk from gaps in current Medicare coverage as well as from certain potential reforms to the program.

5.

QUALITY

Principle V. Medicare should be a responsible steward that works to promote and encourage high quality care and the efficient delivery of medical services.

Medicare has helped bring about major changes in the kind of medical care older and disabled Americans receive and in how and where they receive this care. As the largest single payer for medical services in the United States—and as a dominant payer for many types of services and in some areas of the country—it exercises a greater influence on the health care delivery system than is commonly realized (see Box 5). As a former HCFA administrator points out, the program purchases services in virtually every county and represents "the largest single source of income for the nation's hospitals, physicians, home care agencies, clinical laboratories, durable medical equipment suppliers, and physical and occupational therapists, among others."[1]

In its early years, Medicare was principally, if not exclusively, a financer of care. It paid bills and interacted with the health system largely through its "intermediaries" and "carriers," the health insurance companies that process its day-to-day patient claims. In recent years, Congress and HCFA have taken a more active role in trying to improve the quality and efficiency of health care delivery. This focus has emerged because of new research findings about the health system and the advent of new strategies for financing and delivering care, such as prospective payment and managed care, that have been adopted by private and public payers largely in response to cost pressures. It also reflects a response to evidence that differences in the use

Box 5. How Medicare Has Influenced the Health Care System

Medicare affects the broader health care delivery system in various ways:

- As a payer, it influences providers through what it does and does not cover and by how much it pays for particular procedures and treatments. In 1998, it paid for one out of every five dollars spent on personal health care services, for almost one-third of all payments to hospitals, and for one-quarter of all payments to physicians.

- As a regulator, it sets standards for participation in the program that can determine which institutions operate in a particular county or state and how they practice care. For instance, Medicare's standards for contracting with nursing homes are an industry benchmark, even for those facilities that are not caring for any Medicare-covered patients at a particular time.

- The program also tries to influence the health care system directly by making special payments to hospitals that train doctors and to those that serve an unusually sick population or rural residents.

The original statute authorizing the Medicare program stated that the federal government should not exercise "any supervision or control over the practice of medicine."[a] This "hands-off" posture, reflecting a physicians' consensus that payment for care and hospital administration should be kept separate from the delivery of care, was embedded in the structure of the Blue Cross and Blue Shield plans on which Medicare was modeled.

This conception was already somewhat anachronistic even at Medicare's inception. The program began to influence the broader health care system immediately. One of the first effects was to contribute to the desegregation of southern hospitals. Part A stipulated that Medicare would contract only with hospitals that complied with the provisions of the Civil Rights Act.[b]

The creation of Medicare and Medicaid, somewhat ironically, may have helped facilitate the rapid expansion of for-profit health care corporations. As sociologist Paul Starr points out in *The Social Transformation of American Medicine*, "By making health care lucrative for providers, public financing made it exceedingly attractive to investors and set in motion the formation of large-scale corporate enterprises."[c]

Medicare's coverage and reimbursement policies have stimulated or depressed various sectors of the medical care industry. Congress's decision

(Cont. on the next page)

BOX 5. HOW MEDICARE HAS INFLUENCED
THE HEALTH CARE SYSTEM (CONT.)

to cover treatment for permanent kidney failure boosted the number of kidney dialysis centers, which now receive 95 percent of their revenues from Medicare. In the late 1980s, several legal decisions and coverage rulings greatly expanded eligibility for home health services under Medicare; these services grew from less than 1 percent of total program spending in the late 1960s to 10 percent in 1998.

In the early 1980s, Medicare's relationship to the health care system entered a new phase. If the effects of earlier policies had been largely inadvertent, Congress's decision in 1983 to enact a Prospective Payment System for hospitals—fixed payment per case based on the diagnosis and adjusted by the kind of facility—was designed deliberately to lower Medicare costs and to induce hospital care to be provided more efficiently.[d] PPS had a major impact on how and where Medicare patients received medical treatment.[e] The new reimbursement policies shortened hospital stays and helped usher in a boom in the use of outpatient facilities such as home health agencies and ambulatory surgery centers. By creating excess capacity in hospitals and prompting them to increase prices for private payers, PPS also may have opened the door for HMOs to become price-competitive and gain market share.[f]

[a] From a Generation Behind to a Generation Ahead: Transforming Traditional Medicare, Final Report of the Study Panel on Fee-for-Service Medicare, National Academy of Social Insurance, Washington, D.C., January 1998, p. 14.
[b] Robert M. Ball, "Reflections on How Medicare Came About," in Robert D. Reischauer, Stuart Butler, and Judith R. Lave, eds. Medicare: Preparing for the Challenges of the 21st Century, National Academy of Social Insurance, 1998.
[c] Paul Starr, The Social Transformation of American Medicine: The Rise of a Sovereign Profession and the Making of a Vast Industry (New York: Basic Books, 1984), p. 428.
[d] David G. Smith, Paying for Medicare: The Politics of Reform (Hawthorne, N.Y.: Aldine de Gruyter, 1992), is a superb study of the micropolitics of the development and implementation of hospital—and, later, physician payment—reform.
[e] Some analysts worried that Medicare beneficiaries would be discharged from the hospital "quicker and sicker" as a result of these reforms. The evidence on this question is mixed. One study carried out by the RAND Corporation and UCLA found that the implementation of PPS did not affect observed patient outcomes but that patients were discharged in a less stable condition, which could affect outcomes adversely. It is possible, indeed likely, that other causes were leading to improved outcomes during the period examined by the study. See "Effects of Medicare's Prospective Payment System on the Quality of Hospital Care," Research Highlights, RAND Health, Santa Monica, Calif., 1998, available at http://www.rand.org/publications/RB/RB4519.
[f] Michael L. Millenson, Demanding Medical Excellence: Doctors and Accountability in the Information Age (Chicago: University of Chicago Press, 1997), p. 294.

of medical services are neither necessarily explained by differences in underlying needs nor accompanied by differences in outcomes.[2]

The efforts of legislators and HCFA's staff to improve quality and efficiency in the broader health care delivery system—and thus in the services received by people on Medicare—are commendable. The metaphor of "responsible stewardship" characterizes Medicare's appropriate relationship to these goals. Stewardship suggests Medicare's inevitable involvement in the future of the American health care system. It also conveys the sense of respecting the rights of beneficiaries and looking out for their interests—a goal that prudent innovations promote—as well as of the interests of other stakeholders in Medicare, such as taxpayers and providers. As a public program, however, Medicare needs to move deliberately in the direction of promoting quality and efficiency. This is because of the need to take account of existing statutory requirements and to avoid the possible unintended consequences of reforms.

WHY QUALITY AND VALUE CONCERNS HAVE ARISEN FOR U.S. HEALTH CARE

Concerns about quality of care and the value of the medical services delivered to patients have risen to the fore in recent years. The Institute of Medicine's 1999 estimate that medical errors may result in as many as 98,000 lives lost annually, at a total cost to society of between 17 and 29 billion dollars, for example, drew considerable attention from the media and from researchers.[3] Moreover, the President's Advisory Commission on Consumer Protection and Quality Protection in the Health Care Industry concluded in 1997 that "today, in America, there is no guarantee that any individual will receive high-quality care for any particular health problem. The health care industry is plagued with overutilization of services, underutilization of services, and errors in health care practice."[4] Proposed payment and delivery reforms in the health care system, such as competition among health plans, routinely promise improvements in quality as well as reductions in cost. In practice, financial savings have been easier to gauge and achieve, even when better quality is earnestly sought.

For patient or payer, knowing whether health care is generally of high quality, let alone whether one provider is superior to another, is extremely difficult.[5] As a commodity for purchase, health care is unusual. Patients generally lack—and have found it hard to acquire—the relevant information needed to decide which doctors and treatments to choose. They ordinarily cannot predict when they will be injured or fall ill. Any particular symptom is usually associated with a wide range of possible diagnoses, while a treatment that cures one patient may be ineffective for another. Some patients recover for reasons having nothing to do with the quality of their care, or they die despite receiving state-of-the-art treatment.

Faced with these and many other areas of uncertainty, patients and managers of health benefits have historically turned to doctors for advice and for the coordinated management of treatment. Explicitly and tacitly, patients have traditionally employed a variety of standards as proxies for whether good care is being given: these include the prestige of a hospital or physician, the personal attention they receive, and the ownership structure of a medical institution. [6]

These criteria call attention to the two ways in which quality is currently understood in health care. The first relates to service quality and patient satisfaction with care. The second refers to the technical characteristics of care, especially as reflected in outcomes of treatment or in processes known to affect outcomes. This conception is newer and underlies the movement for quality improvement in medical care that takes its lead from industries such as auto manufacturing (which relies heavily on process measures to support the management theory of "continuous quality improvement"). The technical approach to quality tends to incorporate the idea of efficiency in the way it is defined. For example, one definition characterizes overuse, misuse, and underuse of care as the three primary violations of quality, thus setting the standard of optimal care and the maximization of value as its goal.[7]

From a long-term perspective, this new focus on quality and value has been made possible by the adoption in medicine of scientific standards and procedures, such as the randomized clinical trial, that established the effectiveness of new clinical treatments.[8] Until therapies could be proved to work reliably, the idea that quality of care could be systematically measured and the value of different treatments compared was little more than a visionary's dream.[9]

The more direct causes of this trend toward measuring and evaluating quality involve changes in the way American health care is paid for and practiced. The growth of third-party insurance, spurred by employer coverage for workers after the Second World War and the coverage of the elderly, indigent, and disabled under Medicare and Medicaid in the 1960s, created large organized payers that slowly became interested first in reducing the cost of health benefits and later in the successful treatment of their beneficiaries.

These changes also had an immense impact on the structure and authority of the medical profession. Physicians consolidated their practices. Many joined multispecialty medical groups to cope with the administrative demands of large payers and to keep up with the explosion of relevant clinical knowledge.[10] Specialists proliferated, partly because the coding practices used by insurers gave them an opportunity to maximize their incomes by performing a high volume of procedures. As the collective technical mastery of physicians grew, the number of primary care physicians—traditionally gatekeepers who negotiated entry for patients to the medical system—diminished.

The rise of third-party insurance coverage and the prevalence of fee-for-service payment helped fuel the inflationary trends that characterized both private and public health insurance in the 1970s and early 1980s. Organized payers such as large employers and the government were concerned that the rising costs of health benefits would crimp profits or burden taxpayers. That the Chrysler Corporation paid more for health benefits than for steel entered the popular consciousness. This situation helped to stimulate massive payment reform in Medicare in the mid-1980s and the embrace of managed care by employers in the early 1990s.

In the late 1950s and early 1960s, the late physician and health services researcher Milton Roemer demonstrated that the incidence of hospitalization correlated with the supply of hospital beds in an area.[11] This finding, and others that suggested "induced demand" by physicians, called attention to variability within the health system and to the potential overuse or underuse of medical services. In the early 1970s, John Wennberg and his colleagues demonstrated a similar pattern: the rates of different medical procedures, and the methods by which they were carried out, varied widely from hospital to hospital, town to town, and region to region. Some practice styles did actual harm to patients compared to alternative, preferred treatments; others cost considerably more and appeared to make no difference to the outcome of treatment. Over time, Wennberg compiled a national survey of practice variations.[12] One of the most significant variations, corroborated by a number of studies, was whether beta-blocker drugs were prescribed after patients had suffered heart attacks. While the scientific literature clearly relates this procedure to improved survival rates, a study of hospitals in the state of New Jersey suggested that fewer than one in five patients received this critical treatment.[13]

Findings of this kind have contributed to a new understanding of quality rooted in scientific data as applied to clinical practice. This understanding changed the concept of quality from one principally determined by the judgment of physicians to one susceptible to outside evaluation. Historic relations of trust and deference toward physicians have been affected. Payers for care welcomed the possibility that costs could be lowered while quality remained the same or improved. Prior to congressional passage of hospital prospective payment in Medicare, for example, Wennberg testified to Congress about variations in reimbursement to hospitals under the program, remarking that "the variations suggest opportunities to reduce expenditures under the Medicare and Medicaid programs without reducing the benefits of medical care."[14]

Another important consequence of the increase in insurance coverage, the expansion of government programs, and the consolidation of medical practices is that health care data have become much more comprehensive and readily available. Medicare claims, for example, became the basis for much health services research. While these data still remain fragmentary relative to the ideal of measuring which treatments produce the best health outcomes, they brought the possibility of developing evidence-based measures of quality much closer to reality.

Better data have allowed health care researchers and health administrators to move up the "ladder of quality." However, our ability to measure and improve quality at the level of patient-provider interactions is still seriously hampered by the lack of integrated and sophisticated electronic information systems; the Institute of Medicine, for example, has characterized such systems as essential for achieving this end.[15]

Nevertheless, sufficient progress has been made to allow quality measurement initiatives to develop outcome measures, as well as performance measures that are related to process and structure.[16] Outcomes measures try to judge and compare the end result of particular treatments. Mortality is one outcomes measure; however, many medical procedures are hard to compare on this basis since they rarely result in death. In 1984, for example, Medicare began releasing a pioneering outcome measure, nationwide actual versus expected hospital mortality rates for Medicare patients. This practice was discontinued in 1992 as providers complained that it unfairly discriminated against hospitals that admitted sicker patients.[17] Other important outcome measures include morbidity, which can take into account the number of days a person is unable to perform his or her normal social roles, and maintenance and improvement in functional status and health-related quality of life. QALY (quality-adjusted life year) comparisons, which rely upon surveys of patients' health states and functions, are another form of outcome measure that combines considerations of when people die with how well they live.

Measures of structural quality were among the first developed. They are frequently incorporated into criteria for the accreditation or licensing of health care facilities and providers. The existence of an effective quality assurance system, for example, is often viewed as an important structural measure of quality, as are such indicators as the proportion of doctors on a hospital staff that are board-certified in their speciality or the ratio of nurses to patients in a rehabilitation facility.[18]

Process measures keep track of how regularly a necessary or desirable aspect of treatment is performed, such as administering beta-blockers to heart attack victims. They are often based on the treatment guidelines, protocols, and "clinical pathways" developed and adopted by the government, medical speciality societies, private research groups, and some health plans in an effort to influence provider behavior and to deliver more appropriate care. Process and structural performance measures are expected to serve as proxies for successful outcomes, though the strength of this relationship varies. Often it is more appropriate to view structures and processes as necessary but not sufficient steps to achieving good outcomes.

WHAT MEDICARE DOES AND WHAT IT COULD DO TO IMPROVE THE QUALITY AND EFFICIENCY OF CARE

Payers for health care are now much more actively involved in setting the terms on which health care is delivered and in monitoring its cost and quality. With the consolidation of providers into networks, the ability to collect data on the comparative effectiveness of treatments has grown. The Internet, moreover, offers opportunities for disseminating information on technical quality, and on service satisfaction, much more widely than ever before.[19] These trends have raised hopes that informed third-party payers and individual consumers can raise the quality of the health care system by steering their dollars to health plans and providers that offer the best combination of low cost and expert care. This hope is easy to exaggerate. Many quality measures still link only tenuously to health outcomes.[20] And it is a cliché but true nevertheless that most employers have up to now directed their business to insurers that offer a lower price for health benefits, not high scores on quality measures.

However, progress is beginning to be made in a number of areas—including and in addition to the quality initiatives that Medicare has already undertaken. These activities fall into three broad areas: quality improvement programs that use data collection and assessment methods in an effort to raise the performance of plans and providers, techniques such as selective contracting and disease management, and full-scale value purchasing.

ASSESSING PERFORMANCE AND IMPROVING PROVIDER QUALITY

The first organized effort to boost quality for contractors with Medicare, professional standards review organizations (PSROs), brought together groups of physicians that could make recommendations to withhold Medicare payments to doctors based on evidence of substandard care.[21] They reviewed procedures after the fact, were slow to organize and reluctant to discipline doctors, and had relatively little impact.[22]

Over the life of the program, Medicare's efforts to improve quality of care have evolved from primarily keeping track of structural measures of quality to working actively with providers, Medicare managed care plans, and private organizations in order to develop measures and standards of care. Peer review organizations (PROs), which now monitor fee-for-service Medicare providers and replaced the PSROs in the mid-1980s, have tried more aggressively to improve clinical practices, partly by monitoring providers' success in adhering to process measures of quality.[23]

For example, following national priorities established by HCFA and developed in conjunction with private organizations such as the American Diabetes Association and the Foundation for Accountability, PROs are currently trying to improve the treatment of diabetes, congestive heart failure, acute myocardial infarction, stroke, breast cancer, and pneumonia.[24] Typical process measures for the treatment of diabetes, a disease that afflicts roughly 7 million older Americans, would include the percentage of patients given a foot or eye exam, monitored for kidney disease, and tested for hemoglobin A1c. These efforts appear to be having some effect: one pilot project in four states that assessed progress on heart attack care under these priorities showed overall beta-blocker use increasing from 47 to 68 percent.[25]

HCFA has begun to incorporate performance measurement as a possible criterion for whether it will contract with health plans or hospitals. For instance, a provision in the 1997 Balanced Budget Act stipulated that Medicare managed care plans must demonstrate actual quality improvement in an area important to the health of the population they serve, based on HEDIS (Health Plan-Employer Data and Information Set) measures and CAHPS (Consumer Assessment of Health Plans Study) survey findings (see Box 6). Plans must collect standardized information on various performance measures and on beneficiaries' satisfaction with care. (This is in addition to various structural quality standards that each Medicare+Choice plan must meet, such as maintaining an adequate provider network and observing certain marketing restrictions.[26]) HCFA is also considering using performance measures designed by the Joint Commission on Accreditation of Healthcare Organizations (JCAHO) to monitor the performance of acute care hospitals, with data collection by hospitals becoming a prerequisite for certification by 2003.[27]

To be sure, use of performance measures and standards is controversial. They are vulnerable to the charge that can plausibly be laid against all existing quality measures, namely: Are they meaningful? Do they accurately measure or correlate with the health outcomes that patients and insurers care about? Are they useful? Do they have, or are they likely to have, the effect of improving performance and steering payers and consumers toward higher-quality providers? The application of these performance measures has been heavily weighted toward Medicare+Choice plans, in part because it is conceptually and logistically difficult to generate data on individual fee-for-service providers. Managers of HMOs understandably find this differential burden unfair, noting that they already confront more extensive regulations than insurance companies in most states, including state insurance commission and Medicaid reviews.[28] Because implementing and tracking a single performance measure can cost a plan anywhere

Box 6. HEDIS and CAHPS

HEDIS (Health Plan-Employer Data and Information Set)

About 90 percent of HMOs provide data for HEDIS, a prominent effort to gather comparative information on Medicare managed care plans with the aim of promoting informed purchasing by employers and patients. HEDIS was launched in 1991 by the National Committee on Quality Assurance (NCQA), an organization founded by employers, managed care plans, and nonprofit foundations. It offers quality information about health plans on a variety of clinical and service measures, such as beta-blocker treatment and cholesterol screening after a heart attack, breast cancer screening, and member satisfaction. In 1999, information on all 410 participating plans, evaluated in fifty categories, would have filled the equivalent of four thousand pages of text.[a]

CAHPS (Consumer Assessment of Health Plans Study)

CAHPS is a federally funded project, initiated by the Agency for Health Care Policy and Research in 1996 and administered under cooperative agreements with teams of researchers. The study attempts to develop meaningful consumer assessments of health plans and medical services. It has created standardized surveys that are given to Medicare beneficiaries and privately insured individuals for the purposes of rating their experience and satisfaction with their plans or providers. CAHPS survey findings are part of the HEDIS measurement set, and are becoming increasingly widely used.[b]

[a] See *The State of Managed Care Quality 1999*, National Committee for Quality Assurance, Washington, D.C., 1999; David Dranove, *The Economic Evolution of American Health Care: From Marcus Welby to Managed Care* (Princeton, N.J.: Princeton University Press, 2000), pp. 156–58.
[b] For a more detailed description of CAHPS and other population-based surveys, see Jill Eden, "Measuring Access to Care through Population Based Surveys: Where Are We Now?" *Health Services Research* 33, no. 3, Part II (August 1998): 685–707, as well as numerous articles in *Health Services Research* 36, no. 3, July 2001. See also the CAHPS website, available at http://www.ahcpr.gov/qual/cahpsix.htm.

from $20,000 to $700,000, these managers are concerned when fee-for service providers do not have to meet similar requirements.[29] In this regard, it is noteworthy that a fee-for-service version of CAHPS is now being administered and its findings will be released shortly. Government regulators of Medicare should seek parity among the data collection burdens the program places on plans and fee-for-service providers. Furthermore, since the vast majority of people on Medicare remain in the fee-for-service system, it is essential that improvements be made in the quality of that system, which has recently been found to conform to the pattern of the serious variations in quality reported for the U.S. delivery system overall.[30]

In its 1999 summary of its work, the National Committee for Quality Assurance reported that for the first time health plans that scored higher on performance measures also received higher scores for consumer satisfaction. It also found that plans that had been reporting data for a longer time were scoring higher, a possible demonstration of the positive effects of accountability.[31] Plans are responding to the performance measures incorporated into HEDIS and CAHPS—which increases the pressure on the designers of these measures to be sure they are the best ones available. This development raises hopes that performance accountability in combination with informed purchasing will help lead to actual and important quality improvements.

INNOVATIONS TO MEDICARE FEE-FOR-SERVICE BASED ON MANAGED CARE TECHNIQUES

Managed care plans strive to achieve efficiencies and maintain quality standards by constructing a network of providers and suppliers who accept a plan's payment rules and treatment guidelines. One set of proposed reforms for making Medicare more efficient would adapt methods used by managed care plans to the fee-for-service sector of the program, which currently enrolls about 85 percent of all beneficiaries.

A study panel on fee-for-service Medicare commissioned by the National Academy of Social Insurance recommended that the program consider three specific kinds of strategies: contracting selectively with providers, purchasing medical supplies through a process of competitive procurement, and establishing disease and case management programs.[32] Disease management programs would permit Medicare to contract with and establish new payment rules for providers who specialize in coordinated treatment of certain high-cost chronic conditions; they would introduce incentives as well for patients to learn and use self-care and prevention strategies.

Using these strategies could allow Medicare to steer beneficiaries toward lower-cost, higher-quality providers, potentially raising the value of the services offered for beneficiaries and taxpayers. Former President Clinton's comprehensive Medicare reform proposal of 1999 featured various proposals of this kind, including a plan to make "Centers of Excellence"—providers that specialize in certain high-cost, high-difficulty procedures such as heart bypass surgery—a permanent part of the program, as well as a proposal to lower the cost sharing for Medicare beneficiaries who chose certain providers.[33] This latter proposal resembles in terms of organization the "preferred provider" plans (which now constitute the majority of managed care plans in the employer market) in which policyholders can go outside a network for treatment but pay more out-of-pocket if they do so.

Since most of these strategies are of recent vintage, the evidence of their effectiveness is as yet varied and incomplete. As they evolve and grow in importance, it is vital to ensure that their use is designed and evaluated in terms of improvements in quality rather than just reductions in costs. As a large and public payer that strives to ensure access to good care for all its beneficiaries, Medicare also must be prudent in pursuing policies that might have inadvertent adverse consequences. In some ways, the very size and strength of Medicare as a payer can limit its ability to take steps that would be far more feasible and appropriate, and perhaps advisable, for private payers. For example, deciding to contract selectively with providers that met certain benchmarks for quality rather than employing a lower "threshold of competence" approach might reduce the number of physicians who treat Medicare patients. In some rural areas where Medicare patients represent a large proportion of the caseload, it might jeopardize the livelihood of certain providers, surely an unintended consequence of certain reforms.

VALUE PURCHASING

In recent years, a number of coalitions led by businesses and private foundations have been spearheading efforts to develop innovative ways of identifying and paying for quality care. Many of these coalitions have operated at a local or regional level, such as the Pacific Business Group on Health, the Buyers Health Care Action Group, the Midwest Business Group on Health, and the Central Florida Health

Care Coalition. They often incorporate a mix of private employers—
large, medium, and small—and state and local public sector employers.
Recently, a consortium of Fortune 500 companies and large purchasers, the Leapfrog Group, has been created, largely in response to
concerns about medical errors and patient safety. The Foundation for
Accountability, based in Portland, Oregon, also supports purchaser-
and consumer-oriented initiatives in quality measurement and
improvement. The organization works to develop more clinically rig-
orous, condition-specific sets of performance measures as well as methods for presenting comparisons of health care quality to consumers.[34]

The most important activities of these business coalitions generally
involve collecting and disseminating information and data on quality,
group purchasing on behalf of their employees, and incorporating financial incentives in the contracts they negotiate. In particular, they may hold
a portion of premiums contingent on achievement of certain levels of
performance or performance improvement.[35] In the immediate future,
the first of these activities is the most likely to be relevant to Medicare.[36]

With regard to financial incentives, a Medicare program remod-
eled along premium support lines could theoretically withhold a portion of its premium payment to a plan in return for the plan's meeting
demonstrable quality goals. But this and other efforts to achieve "market accountability" would be difficult to implement given Medicare's
existing fee-for-service orientation and its statutory and political limitations on "deselecting" providers. Value-purchasing efforts are most
likely to succeed when the market for health care providers is competitive and exclusive networks with tighter rules have greater appeal for
providers. Because Medicare, like many employers, operates in many
areas where relatively few providers practice, it often lacks the opportunity to undertake purchasing for value even if it had the authority
and the will to do so. However, in light of the many initiatives devoted
to this end, legislators should be willing to grant Medicare more flexibility to conduct demonstrations under its statute so that it could try to
emulate successful value-purchasing programs that emerge.[37]

CONCLUSION

Medicare should exercise its undoubted influence toward the end
of improving quality and efficiency in health care. The program's
ultimate goal is the health and well-being of its beneficiaries, and it

has a clear responsibility to ensure that the services it offers are at least as high quality and efficient as those received by the average American. In the spirit of responsible stewardship, it must take full advantage of the increasing opportunities to measure and improve quality that have emerged over the past several years.

However, it also has a definite responsibility—grounded in both statute and tradition—to be fair to other stakeholders in the program such as physicians and Medicare+Choice plans. Nor should the difficulty of improving the quality and value of the health care delivery system be underestimated. "Fixing" quality is not simple, primarily because the sources of quality care lie deep in the day-to-day operations of the system itself, and systems are notoriously difficult to change in fundamental and sustainable ways. In addition, the quality agenda will always have to contend with the preoccupation of payers, including government payers, with cost containment rather than value considerations.

Nevertheless, the effort to boost quality through a variety of strategies, including internal quality improvement efforts, more informed purchasing, and greater accountability, is important and useful. Making gains in the value of health care delivered could reduce or delay the need to raise taxes or increase beneficiary cost sharing. As a responsible steward, Medicare should work to ensure that the care that beneficiaries receive is appropriate, of consistently good quality, and of generally high value.

6.

BENEFICIARY EDUCATION AND CHOICE

Principle VI. The process by which people with Medicare choose among alternative health insurance options and products should be made easier: it should clarify important distinctions among different types of health insurance and provide useful and unbiased education, information, and decision support to beneficiaries and those who help them make choices.

The choices made by people with Medicare can affect the extent and quality of health care they receive and the price they pay for it. These important choices include:

- selecting an individual health care provider;

- choosing a group of health care providers;

- selecting a treatment option;

- picking out a health insurance option (e.g., traditional Medicare, Medicare+Choice, Medigap); and

- within Medicare+Choice and Medigap, choosing a specific health plan and product.

The past several years have witnessed an enormous increase in the range of health insurance products potentially available to people on Medicare. Although Medicare remains largely a fee-for-service program, in passing the Balanced Budget Act of 1997, Congress created the Medicare+Choice program, defining choice primarily in terms of *type of health insurance product.* Medicare+Choice not only made several existing types of health insurance products available to people on Medicare (for example, preferred provider plans) but introduced new types of plans never before seen in the health care marketplace (such as private fee-for-service plans).

This legislation, like most health policy over the past several years, assumes that competitive markets ensure both efficiency and effectiveness in health care delivery. A key feature of a competitive market is that buyers have meaningful choices and that they have information they can use to make those choices. There is considerable evidence, however, that providing information to support choice for millions of people on Medicare—who have diverse learning capacities and styles, different menus of choice available according to their specific circumstances, and different health care needs—is a task that will require considerable resources, wise strategies, and a good deal of time to execute effectively.[1]

For the concept of choice to be put into action in a way that both empowers people on Medicare and improves the effectiveness of market-based reforms, it is imperative that reform efforts focus on improving the quality of choices available in all Medicare options—as well as the quality of information available to compare choices. Though making a range of choices available is important, it is just as important that they be meaningful choices from the point of view of consumers. Meaningful implies the distinctiveness of choices, the comprehensibility of choices, and the choice of provider as well as the choice of insurance product and specific plan. It also requires the development of a broader Medicare "information infrastructure" that responds effectively to the varied needs and characteristics of enrollees.

DISTINCTIVENESS OF CHOICES

Given the diversity of the Medicare population, providing a range of health insurance product choices is valuable. However, this value can be diminished if the types of insurance product available are hard for even well-versed policy analysts to distinguish from one another.

For example, for many years specific combinations of supplemental benefits available in the private Medigap market proliferated. Differences between products were often of the "hairsplitting" variety, and it was extremely difficult for people on Medicare to figure out exactly how benefit package differences would affect them if and when they needed health services. In response, Congress legislated a requirement that Medigap plans be limited to a set of ten standardized benefit packages to make it easier for people to choose which set of benefits they would want and to determine which insurance company offered such a benefit package at the lowest premium.

Though differences between types of health plans and insurance products may prove significant in practice, they are often anything but clear-cut. In terms of its potential impact on Medicare beneficiaries, what is the critical distinction between an HMO operated by an insurance company and a provider sponsored organization operated by a group of providers when both face the same financial and market realities? What differentiates two HMOs with almost identical premiums and covered services and an 80 percent overlap in their provider networks? Identifying the meaningful differences and explaining them to people on Medicare represents a significant challenge.

Furthermore, it can be confusing when choices are described that have never been available or are no longer available to people living in a specific market. Under the Balanced Budget Act, Congress permitted Medicare to contract not only with HMOs but with PPOs, PSOs,[2] and with private fee-for-service plans. It also permitted the marketing of medical savings accounts to a limited number of people. Few insurers, have, however, actually offered these new types of products to people on Medicare, at least to date.[3]

The evaluation of HCFA's Medicare Education Program suggests that the vast majority of consumers do not understand what these new products are.[4] A recent study by Judith Hibbard notes that very few people on Medicare understand significant differences between the original fee-for-service program and Medicare HMOs, even though these have been available in some areas for more than fifteen years. Hibbard found, in fact, that those actually enrolled in HMOs were less likely to understand how they differed from fee-for-service Medicare.[5]

It is important to distinguish between options that are theoretically available and those that are both actually available and within the financial reach of the average (that is, moderate-income) person on Medicare. For example, if Medigap plans with significant prescription drug coverage either are not being offered because of biased selection concerns or are priced at unaffordable levels, they will not be perceived as plausible alternatives.

COMPREHENSIBILITY OF CHOICES

Multiplying the sheer number of choices can make the process of selection far more difficult for people on Medicare. By increasing the cognitive complexity involved in comparisons of products with multidimensional characteristics, a proliferation of options can even be perceived as a burden rather than as an asset.[6] Providing information to support choices is made far more difficult when the number of choices gets beyond a certain point. Cognitive psychologists have long known that people can keep about five items, plus or minus two, in their short-term memory at any given point in time. (This is one reason why expert systems designed to provide "decision support" often work by helping people narrow their choices down to facilitate comparisons and trade-offs.) Past a certain point, people will disengage from the effort of consciously choosing. Thus, increasing the number of choices can actually undermine the "choice" strategy and limit the real ability of people covered by Medicare to choose—and perceive that they have chosen—how they will get their health care.

CHOICES OF PROVIDER AND PLAN

Especially in markets where Medicare HMOs are a relatively recent phenomenon, many people on Medicare are less interested in choosing among different types of health insurance products than they are in retaining relatively free choice of specific health plans, specific health care providers, and for some, specific diagnostic and treatment procedures.[7] Indeed, resistance to HMOs is a response not only to perceived limitations in access but to the reality that provider choice will be limited to a defined network.

For some people, concerns over "who is in the network" appear fairly straightforward: they have a good relationship with one (or often several) clinicians, and they do not want to give that up. For others, the roots of the concern are more difficult to entangle, and provider choice may be a proxy for other considerations, such as control or quality. Especially when people have had (or perceive that they have had) complete freedom to choose their doctors and hospitals, giving up that freedom creates nervousness, even when there is little reason to believe that they would actually be able, on their own, to find a better clinician outside the network than those available within the network. Most people, after all, use something like the Yellow Pages at present to choose their primary care doctor and typically leave the selection of specialist to their generalist. This may not be terribly different, operationally, from picking from a plan's provider directory and having their primary care doctor serve as a gatekeeper for specialty care referrals. Many people, however, worry that this approach will make it impossible for them, should they become seriously ill, to find the "best"-quality clinician or facility for their particular condition. This concern is reflected in the efforts of many Medicare HMOs to include highly prestigious medical centers in their networks and also may be a major reason for offering a "point of service" option that gives people the sense that, in a pinch, they could make the decision to use a non-network provider.

To be sure, people on Medicare have expressed concerns regarding the availability, in their geographic region or for people with their health status, of specific plans. The sudden withdrawal of many Medicare HMOs, either completely or from specific markets, led in many cases to dismay from consumers and advocates alike. Many who had questioned the value of such plans were distressed once these were no longer available, largely because they had become an affordable way to acquire prescription benefits and otherwise reduce out-of-pocket expenses without having to pay the extremely high premiums increasingly required for the high-end Medigap plans. Even in this context, however, it is fairly clear that people were not concerned about the overall number of plans from which they could choose but rather worried about whether they could keep a particular plan (the one they had) or get another plan that was as similar to it as possible, especially in terms of costs and coverage.

BUILDING AN EFFECTIVE INFORMATION INFRASTRUCTURE

Perhaps the most important imperative is to provide useful and unbiased education, comparative data, and decision support, so that choices can and will be well informed rather than random. For the population served by the Medicare program, this is not an easy task. A substantial fraction of people on Medicare are cognitively impaired or otherwise far too frail to make health plan comparisons on their own. The general literacy and numeracy levels of this population are quite low, making it difficult if not impossible for the vast majority to comprehend accurately text written at more than sixth-grade level, a simple comparison table, or more fundamentally the complexities involved in choosing a health plan or provider.[8]

In addition, baseline understanding of the traditional Medicare program is and always has been fairly low[9] (see Figure 17). HCFA historically has put few resources or expertise into "beneficiary awareness." It does not have a nationwide network of district offices available to people across the country, like those of the Social Security Administration, which can provide information and assistance to people on Medicare. The government has supported—at an extremely low level given the size of the population served ($10 million per year prior to Balanced Budget Act, when it was increased to $15 million)—state programs to provide information, counseling, and assistance to people with regard to their questions about Medicare, Medigap, and Medicare HMOs. Several states supplement these resources with their own. Nevertheless, this State Health Insurance Information Program (SHIP) has only a limited capacity to provide personal assistance to the millions of people on Medicare who have questions and problems.

In the Balanced Budget Act, Congress assigned an extensive series of beneficiary education tasks to HCFA. Legislators specified what kinds of comparative data should be presented and how these data were to be disseminated (including an annual mailing of the *Medicare & You Handbook*, a hotline 1-800–MEDICARE number, and a website called www.medicarecompare.gov). These mandates have galvanized HCFA to generate meaningful comparative data about options and to provide these data, along with extensive background information about the program, in a consistent manner. While HCFA has made considerable progress in these tasks, it is still some way from the goal of providing useful and unbiased information

FIGURE 17. HOW MUCH AMERICANS SAY THEY KNOW ABOUT MEDICARE AND REFORM OPTIONS FOR MEDICARE (SURVEY CONDUCTED AUGUST–SEPTEMBER 1998)

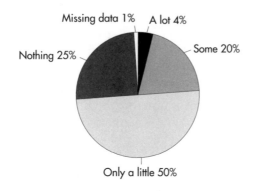

Missing data 1%   A lot 4%

Nothing 25%   Some 20%

Only a little 50%

Source: National Survey on Medicare, Henry J. Kaiser Family Foundation/Harvard School of Public Health, Washington, D.C., October 28, 1998, Chart 8, available at http://www.kff.org/content/archive/1442/reform_cp.pdf.

to everyone who needs it.[10] Increasingly, experts in consumer information and decisionmaking agree that, in addition to meaningful educational materials, an information infrastructure is needed to provide personal assistance to people on Medicare as they learn to navigate the complexities of the current and emerging health market. In particular, experts believe it is essential to tailor information to meet the needs of subpopulations defined by characteristics such as language, culture, health status, literacy level, and region of residence. Most efforts to date have emphasized creating generic products for "all" people on Medicare. Tailoring has occurred largely at the local level, with little if any support from HCFA.

In addition, the resource base for the educational efforts is uncertain. Under the Balanced Budget Act, Medicare+Choice plans were assigned the responsibility for financing the provision of comparative data. Dismayed by this burden and further distressed that at the outset comparative quality data were available only on HMOs rather than on all options, including the fee-for-service program, the plans successfully lobbied to reduce their payments in support of the Medicare Education Program. In the short term, money has come from the trust fund, but this is not an appropriate or sustainable source for the middle to long term.

If the "choice" strategy is to be effective, for individual beneficiaries, for the Medicare program as a whole, and for the health care delivery system, it is essential that stable resources be provided to support efforts to improve the quality of data available for comparing health plans and health care providers. This entails:

- providing data not only on HMOs but also on the original Medicare program and other, newer health insurance plan options as well; HCFA is already beginning to "level the playing field" by providing quality data on the fee-for-service program—these efforts need to be sustained and deepened;

- providing data that are more easily viewed as salient by consumers[11] (see Figure 18);

- providing data to help people compare medical groups, hospitals, nursing homes, and other providers as well as health insurance plans;

- supporting the development of information systems for plans and providers that will make data collection less burdensome.[12]

The choice strategy also depends on efforts to measure and improve the effectiveness of consumer education and decision support efforts, namely:

- continuing efforts to develop and test innovative as well as traditional approaches to providing information to people on Medicare, including approaches that take into consideration differences in language, culture, and literacy;[13]

- building a stable infrastructure that enables people on Medicare, and those who help them make choices, to get tailored and personalized assistance.

By facilitating the process by which people on Medicare choose among different health insurance products, these measures will widen the range and enhance the quality of medical services they receive while making the health care system more efficient.

FIGURE 18. HOW MANY BENEFICIARIES CONSIDERED CHANGING THEIR HEALTH CARE COVERAGE, 2000

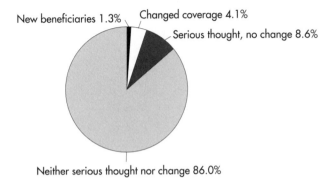

New beneficiaries 1.3%   Changed coverage 4.1%

Serious thought, no change 8.6%

Neither serious thought nor change 86.0%

Source: Marsha Gold and Natalie Justh, "How Salient Is Choice to Medicare Beneficiaries?" *Monitoring Medicare and Choice Fast Facts* no. 5, Princeton, N.J., January 2001.

7.

ADMINISTRATION

Principle VII. Medicare's management and administrative capac-
ities should be adequately funded so that the goals implied by
these principles can be carried out effectively in the context of a
growing Medicare population.

A major theme of this report is that Medicare needs more
resources to succeed, both now and in the future. Facing a surge in
beneficiaries in less than a decade, a rise in the number of useful
medical therapies, and a benefit package that lags behind the private sector norm, Medicare spending needs to increase if the program's original promise—access to high-quality medical care and
protection from financial ruin for the elderly and disabled—is to
be fulfilled.

With these broad aims in mind, legislators should devote more
resources to the program's management and administration. Current
funding levels are inadequate to the number of beneficiaries that the
program serves—and will serve. They also are inadequate for carrying
out the operational tasks that the program's managers are being called
upon or may be called upon, to implement (see Figure 19, page 102).[1]

When responsibility for Medicare was shifted away from the
Social Security Administration to the newly formed Health Care
Financing Administration in 1977, the agency had a staff of 4,000.
Almost twenty-five years later, the staff size has remained virtually the
same, even though the number of beneficiaries has grown from 26
million to 39 million and program spending is 3.6 times greater in
real dollars (see Figure 20, page 102).

FIGURE 19. TRENDS IN ADMINISTRATIVE
COST AS PERCENTAGE OF BENEFITS

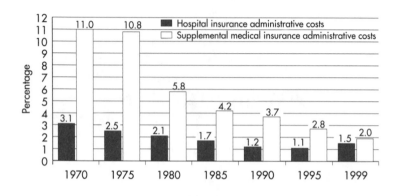

Source: U.S. Congress, House Committee on Ways and Means, May 17, 1999, Figure 3.28.

FIGURE 20. SMI AND HI FUND EXPENDITURES AND
ADMINISTRATION COST, IN BILLIONS OF DOLLARS

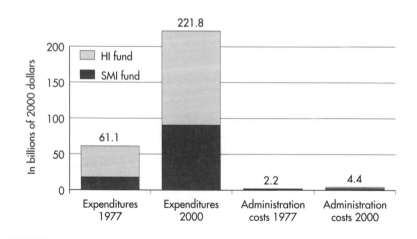

Note: Changes from 1977 to 2000: 3.6 times increase in expenditures; 2.0 times increase in admnistration costs.
Source: Annual Report of the Board of Trustees of the Federal Hospital Insurance Trust Fund and Annual Report of the Board of Trustees of the HI and SMI Trust Funds.

In the meantime, in addition to processing a larger number of claims, the number of tasks that the agency has been called on to perform has mushroomed. Medicare and Medicaid rules, as published in the *Federal Register*, have proliferated in the past decade in response to congressional mandates. (The Mayo Foundation has estimated that one large midwestern hospital is affected by 132,720 pages of Medicare and Medicaid rules alone.[2]) Under legislation such as the Health Insurance Portability and Accountability Act of 1996 and the Balanced Budget Act of 1997, Medicare's administrators were charged with introducing Medicare+Choice, responding to Y2K readiness issues, making the agency more consumer-friendly, and beefing up the enforcement of antifraud provisions. Should they take a more active role in ensuring that providers and plans are accountable for quality, as a previous section of this report discussed, their duties will expand even further.

As a diverse group of stakeholders and policy experts explained in a 1999 open letter to Congress, "The mismatch between the agency's administrative capacity and its political mandate has grown enormously over the 1990s. . . . The sheer complexity of its new policy directives is mind-boggling and requires a new generation of employees with the requisite skills. HCFA's ability to provide assistance to beneficiaries, monitor the quality of provider services, and protect against fraud and abuse has been increasingly compromised by the failure to provide the agency with adequate administrative resources."[3]

Regulations often produce their intended results. The large reduction in Medicare overpayments brought about by new antifraud measures is a case in point. More generally, detailed regulations protect taxpayers and beneficiaries from fraud and ensure that contractors and providers know their responsibilities and are paid fairly.[4]

However, new regulations can be burdensome for physicians, health plans, and postacute care facilities. These providers express concerns about slow and inconsistent decisionmaking by HCFA and contractors that process Medicare claims, about unrealistic demands for data to satisfy quality improvement initiatives, about insufficient notice of new regulations, and about lack of guidance about how to comply with newly implemented rules. While these problems may diminish as regulators and providers become more accustomed to new rules, it is clear that compliance with even well-intended regulations may conflict sharply with the mission of caring for patients.[5]

Making more resources available might allow the program's administration to take steps toward alleviating these burdens. For example, intermediaries and carriers—the private insurers that handle most of Medicare's day-to-day interactions with individual providers and beneficiaries—could receive substantial additional funds to improve their capacity to explain new rules and coverage decisions to providers. More judges who specialize in adjudicating Medicare claims made by providers and beneficiaries could be hired.[6]

To be sure, improving Medicare's administration is not simply a question of increasing the program's funding. Many proposals to modernize and streamline Medicare's management have been offered in recent years.[7] To take just one example, oversight of Medicaid and the State Children's Health Insurance Program (S-CHIP) might be transferred out of HCFA to another agency, freeing up HCFA's staff to focus solely on managing Medicare. Assessing the potential advantages and disadvantages of particular proposals for administrative reform goes beyond the scope of this report.[8] However, a sound overhaul of Medicare will depend on the availability of more resources for managing the program, regardless of which administrative reforms are eventually adopted.

NOTES

INTRODUCTION

1. *National Survey on Medicare*, Henry J. Kaiser Family Foundation/Harvard School of Public Health, Washington, D.C., October 28, 1998, Chart 1, available at http://www.kff.org/content/archive/1442/reform_cp.pdf.

2. Cathy Schoen et al., *Counting on Medicare: Perspectives and Concerns of Americans Ages 50 to 70,* Commonwealth Fund, New York, July 2000.

3. See Senator John Breaux (D.-La.), quoted in the transcript on the website of the National Bipartisan Commission on the Future of Medicare, available at http://thomas.loc.gov/medicare/tran3698.html.

4. For definitions of social insurance, see, in particular, *Medicare and the American Social Contract,* Final Report of the Study Panel on Medicare's Larger Social Role, National Academy of Social Insurance, Washington, D.C., February 1999; Michael J. Graetz and Jerry L. Mashaw, *True Security: Rethinking American Social Insurance* (New Haven: Yale University Press, 1999).

5. Robert B. Friedland, "Privatization and Public Policy," *Public Policy and Aging Report* 9, no. 2 (1998), National Academy on an Aging Society, Washington, D.C., p. 10.

6. Cf. Mark McClellan, "Medicare Reform: Fundamental Problems, Incremental Steps," *Journal of Economic Perspectives* 14, no. 2 (Spring 2000): 21–44.

7. In fact, each of the thirteen significant reforms to Medicare enacted between 1982 and 1997 was carried out through legislation aimed at reducing budget deficits.

8. Annual Report of the Board of Trustees of the Federal Hospital Insurance Trust Fund, 2001, available at http://www.hcfa.gov/pubforms/tr/default.htm.

9. Rudolph Penner, "Money, Money Everywhere," *Milken Institute Review*, Second Quarter 2000, p. 4.

10. McClellan, "Medicare Reform."

11. *Demography Is Not Destiny*, National Academy on an Aging Society, Washington, D.C., January 1999, p. 27.

12. See David Cutler, "Walking the Tightrope on Medicare Reform," *Journal of Economic Perspectives* 14, no. 2 (Spring 2000): 45–56; James Lubitz et al., "Three Decades of Health Care Use by the Elderly, 1965–1998," *Health Affairs* 20, no. 2 (March/April 2001): 19–32; Charles R. Morris, *Too Much of a Good Thing? Why Health Care Spending Won't Make Us Sick* (New York: The Century Foundation Press, 2000).

13. Kenneth G. Manton, Larry Corder, and Eric Stallard, "Chronic Disability Trends in Elderly United States Populations: 1982–1994," *Proceedings of the National Academy of Sciences* 94 (1997), argue that disabilities among the elderly are declining.

14. See "Medicare's Experience with Competitive Pricing," special section, *Health Affairs* 19, no. 5 (September/October 2000): 6–59.

15. See especially Cara S. Lesser and Paul B. Ginsburg, "Back to the Future? New Cost and Access Challenges Emerge," CSHSC Issue Brief no. 35, Center for Studying Health System Change, Washington, D.C., February 2001.

16. Stephen Heffler et al., "Health Spending Growth Up in 1999; Faster Growth Expected in the Future," *Health Affairs* 20, no. 2 (March/April 2001): 193–203. A substantial literature debates whether managed care poses special difficulties for frail and disabled Medicare beneficiaries. Richard Kronick and Joy de Beyer, *Medicare HMOs: Making Them Work for the Chronically Ill* (Chicago: Health Administration Press, 1998), is a good summary of the differing views.

17. Institute of Medicine, *Crossing the Quality Chasm: A New Health System for the 21st Century* (Washington, D.C.: National Academy Press, 2001).

18. By reason of custom and statute, Medicare has historically been reluctant to "interfere in the practice of medicine." Though this proscription is increasingly vestigial, it continues to constrain direct efforts by the program to improve the quality and efficiency of the medical delivery system.

19. Jonathan Skinner, "Medicare Reform: Improving Fairness and Efficiency," Center for Evaluative Clinical Sciences, Dartmouth Medical School, n.d., available at http://www.dartmouthatlas.org/medicarereform/medicare_reform.php.

20. On June 14, 2001, this agency was renamed the Centers for Medicare and Medicaid Services (CMS).

21. Health Care Financing Administration, *A Profile of Medicare: Chart Book*, May 1998; U.S. Congress, House, Committee on Ways and Means, *Medicare and Health Care Chartbook*, May 17, 1999.

CHAPTER 1

1. Social Security—which pays for a modest pension that partially replaces the prior earnings of older and disabled Americans—and Medicare are the largest and most popular U.S. social insurance programs. For a succinct

description and analysis of the concept and practice of social insurance, see Harvey S. Rosen, *Public Finance*, 4th ed. (Homewood, Ill.: Richard D. Irwin, 1995), pp. 195–236.

2. Michael J. Graetz and Jerry L. Mashaw, *True Security: Rethinking American Social Insurance* (New Haven: Yale University Press, 1999), p. 26.

3. Unlike Social Security, the income to which payroll tax contributions apply is not capped at a particular level, meaning that Medicare's financing is more progressive.

4. About 95 percent of those eligible for the program elect to enroll in Part B.

5. As one economic historian puts it, "Whereas the receipt of a relief payment suggested humiliating dependence on the government, the receipt of a social insurance benefit suggested merely the fulfillment of an obligation which had been properly paid for in advance." David A. Moss, "Government, Markets, and Uncertainty: An Historical Approach to Public Risk Management in the United States," working paper, Division of Research, Harvard Business School, 1996.

6. *National Survey on Medicare*, Henry J. Kaiser Family Foundation/Harvard School of Public Health, Washington, D.C., October 28, 1998, available at http://www.kff.org/ content/archive/1442/.

7. Henry J. Kaiser Family Foundation/Harvard School of Public Health/Princeton Survey Research Associates, Post-Election Survey of Voters' 1997 Health Care Agenda, January 1997, quoted in Robert D. Reischauer, Stuart Butler, and Judith R. Lave, eds., *Medicare: Preparing for the Challenges of the 21st Century* (Washington, D.C.: National Academy of Social Insurance, 1998), p. 305.

8. Ibid., p. 311. A recent Henry J. Kaiser Family Foundation/Harvard School of Public Health survey, The Public and the Health Care Agenda for the New Administration and Congress, Washington, D.C., January 25, 2001, finds majority support among the public at large for relating premiums for Medicare to the income of the elderly and for a version of plan choice that resembles premium support.

9. Adverse selection occurs because potential subscribers know more about their need for care than do insurers. At any premium, therefore, an insurance policy will be most attractive to the worst risks and least attractive to the best risks.

10. Theodore R. Marmor, *The Politics of Medicare*, 2d ed. (Hawthorne, N.Y.: Aldine de Gruyter, 2000), p. 13.

11. U.S. Congress, House, Committee on Ways and Means, *2000 Green Book* (Washington, D.C.: U.S. Government Printing Office, 2000), p. 102, Table 2-2. People with disabilities who qualify for Social Security disability payments must wait two years before they qualify for Medicare coverage. For a summary of the characteristics of Medicare's disabled population, and the special challenges facing them, see Marsha Gold and Beth Stevens,

"Medicare's Less Visible Population: Disabled Beneficiaries under Age 65," *Monitoring Medicare+Choice: Operational Insights,* no. 2, Mathematica Policy Research, Princeton, N.J., May 2001.

12. Health Care Financing Administration, *A Profile of Medicare: Chart Book,* May 1998, p. 17, Figure 10.

13. In 1996, 50.4 percent of all Medicare enrollees had payments made on their behalf of less than $500, accounting for just 1.3 percent of total payments, while more than 20 percent had no FFS payments made on their behalf. *Health Care Financing Review: Statistical Supplement,* Health Care Financing Administration, 1998, p. 41, Figure 12.

14. Marilyn Moon, "Growth in Medicare Spending: What Will Beneficiaries Pay?" Commonwealth Fund, New York, May 1999.

15. To be sure, Medicare limits the length of covered hospital stays and lacks "stop-loss" protections on out-of-pocket spending, making it less than true catastrophic protection.

16. As Theodore Marmor writes, "While slightly more than half the persons over 65 had some kind of health insurance in 1962, only 38 percent of the aged no longer working had any insurance at all." Furthermore, surveys of elderly people *with* insurance who had spent time in the hospital found that insurance ended up covering only a small fraction of this most expensive of health care costs.

17. See Joseph Newhouse, "Medical Costs: How Much Welfare Loss?" *Journal of Economic Perspectives* 6, no. 3 (Summer 1992): 11.

18. *Medicare and the American Social Contract,* Final Report of the Study Panel on Medicare's Larger Social Role, National Academy of Social Insurance, Washington, D.C., February 1999, pp. 31–34.

19. A proposal to raise the eligibility age for Medicare passed the House during debate over the Balanced Budget Act of 1995; the National Bipartisan Commission on the Future of Medicare also broached the idea during its deliberations. Much of the rationale for increasing the age of eligibility comes from the comparison between the Medicare eligibility age and the Social Security retirement age, which was in fact increased in 1983 (to take full effect in 2011) from sixty-five to sixty-seven. Yet increasing the Social Security retirement age is essentially the same as cutting benefit levels because retirees as young as sixty-two can obtain reduced Social Security benefits. Raising the eligibility age for Medicare, by contrast, would leave most of those who retire at sixty-five without any source of public coverage (the principal exception would be those unhealthy enough to qualify as disabled or poor enough to receive Medicaid). In response, it has been suggested that a Medicare "buy-in" option could offset whatever negative effects an increase in the age of eligibility for Medicare might have. This is not true of current buy-in proposals, which would charge very high premiums and thus reach very few Americans without private coverage. If the

eligibility age were raised, those most likely to end up uninsured would be precisely the middle- and lower-income Americans who would be unable to afford such premiums.

20. Some people get group coverage from their own or a spouse's former employer, but the availability and sometimes the benefits of these policies are going down, while the retiree contributions are going up, as noted in Chapter 4.

21. Available evidence indicates that if the eligibility age were raised to sixty-seven, more than a third of Americans aged sixty-five to sixty-seven would end up uninsured or severely underinsured, most of them in poor health and with low incomes. Even as it reduced coverage, this change would raise a relatively small amount of new revenue, cutting the total number of Americans eligible for Medicare by more than 11 percent but reducing program costs by only as much as 6.2 percent. Timothy A. Waidmann, "Potential Effects of Raising Medicare's Eligibility Age," *Health Affairs* 17, no. 2 (March/April 1998): 156–63.

22. The rules of the commission stipulated that a supermajority of commissioners was necessary for making formal recommendations, a standard that the group was unable to attain.

23. The history of Medicare contracting strongly indicates that adverse selection is a problem that must be reckoned with if Medicare is to rely more heavily on private health plans. Considerable evidence collected in the 1980s and early 1990s shows that private health plans that contract with Medicare have tended to enroll healthier-than-average beneficiaries, leaving the traditional Medicare program with an adverse selection of risks. See Richard Kronick and Joy de Beyer, *Medicare HMOs: Making Them Work for the Chronically Ill* (Chicago: Health Administration Press, 1998).

24. Ibid.

25. Bruce N. Davidson, Shoshanna Sofaer, and Paul Gertler, "Consumer Information and Biased Selection in the Demand for Coverage Supplementing Medicare," *Social Science and Medicine* 34 (May 1992): 1023–34.

CHAPTER 2

1. For a summary and comparison of how budget specialists have analyzed Medicare's fiscal situation over the past several years, see *Budget Options*, Congressional Budget Office, February 2001, available at http://www.cbo.gov/showdoc.cfm?index=2731&sequence=0&from=1; *Long-term Budgetary Pressures and Policy Options*, Congressional Budget Office, May 1998, available at http://www.cbo.gov/showdoc.cfm?index=492&sequence=0&from=1.

2. Annual Report of the Board of Trustees of the Federal Hospital Insurance Trust Fund, 2001, available at http://www.hcfa.gov/pubforms/tr/default.htm.

3. Part B has always been funded substantially through general revenues. Originally, the amount of the premium was set at 50 percent of Part B costs, a percentage that quickly became onerous for beneficiaries. In the early 1970s, legislation ensured that premium increases would not exceed the cost of living adjustments in Social Security. In the early 1980s, annually renewed legislation set the beneficiary share of premiums at 25 percent of Part B costs. The Balanced Budget Act of 1997 included provisions intended to make this arrangement permanent.

4. The current outlook for the Hospital Insurance Trust Fund is far more optimistic than it was just a few years ago. As recently as in 1996 and 1997 it was estimated that the trust fund would be insolvent in 2001. The 2001 estimate of a 2029 exhaustion date is a significant improvement over the estimate of 2025 made in 2000.

5. David Gross and Normandy Brangan, "Out-of-Pocket Health Spending by Medicare Beneficiaries Age 65 and Older: 1999 Projections," Public Policy Institute, AARP, Washington, D.C., December 1999, p. 1, available at http://research.aarp.org/health/inb14_spend.html.

6. Marilyn Moon, "Growth in Medicare Spending: What Will Beneficiaries Pay?" Commonwealth Fund, New York, May 1999, p. 9, Chart 4.

7. Ibid., p. 11, Chart 6.

8. The 2000 federal poverty guideline is $8350 for an individual, $11,250 for a couple.

9. U.S. Department of Commerce, Bureau of the Census, *Current Population Survey*, figures available at http://www.agingstats.gov/chart-book2000/tables-economics.html#Indicator 7, Table 7.

10. Marilyn Moon, "Beneath the Averages: An Analysis of Medicare and Private Expenditures," Urban Institute, Washington, D.C., September 1999.

11. Michael Gluck and Marilyn Moon, eds., *Financing Medicare's Future*, Final Report of the Study Panel on Medicare's Long Term Financing, National Academy of Social Insurance, Washington, D.C., September 2000, executive summary.

12. Joseph White, "Understanding Long-Term Medicare Cost Estimates," white paper, The Century Foundation, New York, 1999, p. 39.

13. This, indeed, was true of the 1999 Breaux-Frist proposal: average beneficiary premiums would have equaled 12 percent of national per capita Medicare costs when the proposal was fully implemented in 2003, but under current law the Medicare Part B premium is projected to equal only 9.8 of costs in 2003. Gluck and Moon, *Financing Medicare's Future*, Chapter 2.

14. Jill Bernstein, "Should Higher Income Beneficiaries Pay More for Medicare?" Medicare Brief no. 2, National Academy of Social Insurance, Washington, D.C., May 1999.

15. National Academy of Social Insurance analysis based on Barbara Gage et al., "Medicare Savings: Options and Opportunities," discussion paper, Urban Institute, Washington, D.C., June 1997. See also Bernstein, "Should Higher Income Beneficiaries Pay More For Medicare?" note 25.

CHAPTER 3

1. These benefits often include prescription drug coverage and "stop-loss" protection against very large medical expenses incurred in a given year. Health Care Financing Administration, *A Profile of Medicare: Chart Book*, May 1998, p. 3. The original study was conducted by Hewitt Associates and cited in *Medicare Chart Book*, Henry J. Kaiser Family Foundation, Washington, D.C., June 1997. To be sure, some of these employer plans may have added higher copayments, raised premiums, and scaled down their benefit packages in the interim since this study was conducted. For the most up-to-date information on trends in the employer market, see the annual survey conducted by the Henry J. Kaiser Family Foundation and the Health Research Educational Trust, available at http://www.kff.org.

2. On the evolution of the pharmaceutical industry, the process of bringing a drug to market, and the structure of the international marketplace for prescription drugs, see John Mann, *The Elusive Magic Bullet: The Search for the Perfect Drug* (Oxford: Oxford University Press, 1999); Jürgen Drews, *In Quest of Tomorrow's Medicines: An Eminent Scientist Talks about the Pharmaceutical Industry, Biotechnology, and the Future of Drug Research* (New York: Springer-Verlag, 1999); *How Increased Competition from Generic Drugs Has Affected Prices and Returns in the Pharmaceutical Industry*, Congressional Budget Office, July 1998; Stephane Jacobzone, "Pharmaceutical Policies in OECD Countries: Reconciling Social and Industrial Goals," Labor Market and Social Policy—Occasional Papers no. 40, Organization for Economic Co-operation and Development, Paris, April 18, 2000; "Pharmaceutical Marketplace Dynamics," Issue Brief no. 755, National Health Policy Forum, George Washington University, May 31, 2000. On previous discussion of a possible drug benefit for Medicare, begin with Stephen H. Long, "Prescription Drugs and the Elderly: Issues and Options," *Health Affairs* 13, no. 2 (Spring 1994): 157–74. Future projections of chronic illnesses are summarized in a series of briefs issued by the National Academy on an Aging Society, *Data Profiles: Chronic and Disabling Conditions*, especially no.11, "Alzheimer's Disease and Dementia," National Academy on an Aging Society, Washington, D.C., September 2000.

3. Bruce Stuart, Dennis Shea, and Becky Briesacher, "Prescription Drug Costs for Medicare Beneficiaries: Coverage and Health Status Matter," issue brief no. 365, Commonwealth Fund, New York, January 2000, available at http://www.cmwf.org/programs/medfutur/stuart_drug_ib_365.asp.

4. Beth Fuchs et al., *Analyzing Options to Cover Prescription Drugs for Medicare Beneficiaries*, Henry J. Kaiser Family Foundation, Washington, D.C., July 2000, p. 3.

5. U.S. Department of Health and Human Services, *Report to the President: Prescription Drug Coverage, Spending, Utilization, and Prices*, April 2000, p. 40, available at http://aspe.hhs.gov/health/reports/drugstudy/.

6. Cathy Schoen et al., "Counting on Medicare: Perspectives and Concerns of Americans Ages 50 to 70," Commonwealth Fund, New York, July 2000, p. 18.

7. See John A. Poisal and Lauren Murray, "Growing Differences between Medicare Beneficiaries with and without Drug Coverage," *Health Affairs* 20, no. 2 (March/April 2001): 77; John A. Poisal and George S. Chulis, "Medicare Beneficiaries and Drug Coverage," *Health Affairs* 19, no. 2 (March/April 2000): 248.

8. Stuart, Shea, and Briesacher, "Prescription Drug Costs for Medicare Beneficiaries," p. 2; Bruce Stuart, Dennis Shea, and Becky Briesacher, "Dynamics in Drug Coverage of Medicare Beneficiaries: Finders, Losers, Switchers," *Health Affairs* 20, no. 2 (March/April 2001): 86–99. These studies, like those undertaken by Poisal and Chulis, analyze numbers taken from the Medicare Current Beneficiary Survey.

9. Schoen et al., "Counting on Medicare," p. 52.

10. *Prescription Drug Trends: A Chartbook*, Henry J. Kaiser Family Foundation, Washington, D.C., July 2000, p. 6.

11. Margaret Davis et al., "Prescription Drug Coverage, Utilization, and Spending among Medicare Beneficiaries," *Health Affairs* 18, no. 1 (January/February 1999): 241.

12. Poisal and Murray "Growing Differences between Medicare Beneficiaries," p. 82. For additional data, see U.S. Department of Health and Human Services, *Report to the President: Prescription Drug Coverage*, Chapter 2, p. 39. See also David Gross and Normandy Brangan, "Out-of-Pocket Health Spending by Medicare Beneficiaries Age 65 and Older: 1999 Projections," Public Policy Institute, AARP, Washington, D.C., December 1999, available at http://research.aarp.org/health/inb14_spend.html. Disabled Americans take more prescriptions than seniors (about twenty-eight annually), spend more on drugs (an estimated 10 percent of the disabled have more than $2500 in annual spending), and pay more out-of-pocket, according to a White House report. "Disability, Medicare, and Prescription Drugs," National Economic Council and Domestic Policy Council, July 31, 2000.

13. "Medicare and Prescription Drugs," fact sheet, Henry J. Kaiser Family Foundation, Washington, D.C., May 2001, based on CBO estimates. For an earlier estimate, see "A CBO Analysis of the Administration's Prescription Drug Proposal," statement of Dan L. Crippen, director, Congressional

Budget Office, before the Subcommittee on Health, U.S. Congress, House, Committee on Ways and Means, 106th Cong., 2d sess., May 11, 2000.

14. U.S. Department of Health and Human Services, *Report to the President: Prescription Drug Coverage*, p. 96. The difference is 15 percent on average at a minimum and would presumably be higher if rebates commonly granted to insurers were factored in.

15. Stuart, Shea, and Briesacher, "Prescription Drug Costs for Medicare Beneficiaries," pp. 5–6. Because those individuals who need to use prescription drugs are most likely to purchase coverage, it is hard to link improved health status directly to greater drug use. This study showed that beneficiaries with multiple chronic illnesses are in fact more likely to have steady coverage than those who are in good health.

16. Jan Blustein, "Drug Coverage and Drug Purchases by Medicare Beneficiaries with Hypertension," *Health Affairs* 19, no. 2 (March/April 2000): 224.

17. Poisal and Murray, "Growing Differences between Medicare Beneficiaries," p. 80. In this study, beneficiaries without insurance below the poverty line took 13.7 fewer prescriptions annually than their insured counterparts; for those beneficiaries with incomes exceeding 400 percent of poverty, this gap narrowed to 3.86 prescriptions per year.

18. Paul Grootendorst et al., "On Becoming 65 in Ontario: Effects of Drug Plan Eligibility on Use of Prescription Medicines," *Medical Care* 35, no. 4 (April 1997): 386–98.

19. "Still Rising: Drug Price Increases for Seniors 1999–2000," Families USA, Washington, D.C., April 2000. See also the earlier report, "Hard to Swallow: Rising Drug Prices for America's Seniors," Families USA, Washington, D.C., November 1999.

20. Marsha Gold, "Trends Reflect Fewer Choices," *Monitoring Medicare+Choice: Fast Facts*, no. 4, Mathematica Policy Research, Princeton, N.J., September 2000.

21. June Gibbs Brown, "HMO Withdrawals: Impact on Medicare Beneficiaries," memorandum, U.S. Department of Health and Human Services, August 2000.

22. Marsha Gold and Natalie Justh, "Forced Exit: Beneficiaries in Plans Terminating in 2000," *Monitoring Medicare+Choice: Fast Facts*, no. 3, Mathematica Policy Research, Princeton, N.J., September 2000; "Medicare HMOs Serve Many Financially Vulnerable Beneficiaries," *Facts & Figures*, American Association of Health Plans, Washington, D.C., May 17, 2000.

23. "The Implications of Medicare Prescription Drug Proposals for Employers and Retirees," report prepared by Frank McCardle et al., Hewitt Associates LLC, for the Henry J. Kaiser Family Foundation, Washington, D.C., July 2000.

24. Laura Dummitt, "Medigap: Premiums for Standardized Plans that Cover Prescription Drugs," letter to John D. Dingell, U.S. Congress, House,

Committee on Commerce, March 1, 2000. See also Michael E. Gluck, "A Medicare Prescription Drug Benefit," Medicare Brief no.1, National Academy of Social Insurance, Washington, D.C., April 1999.

25. "The Role of PBMs in Managing Drug Costs: Implications for a Medicare Drug Benefit," report prepared by Anna Cook, Thomas Kornfield, and Marsha Gold, Mathematica Policy Research, for the Henry J. Kaiser Family Foundation, Washington, D.C., January 2000, p. 24.

26. Because the time that a drug is in clinical trials is included in its term of patent protection, some believe that the effective period during which pharmaceutical companies can turn a profit on a new drug and try to recoup their R&D costs is compressed, and may have become more so. See *How Increased Competition from Generic Drugs Has Affected Prices and Returns in the Pharmaceutical Industry,* Congressional Budget Office, July 1998.

27. "Factors Affecting the Growth of Prescription Drug Expenditures," report prepared by Barents Group LLC for the National Institute for Health Care Management Research and Educational Foundation, Washington, D.C., July 9, 1999, p. 12-14; U.S. Department of Health and Human Services, *Report to the President: Prescription Drug Coverage,* p. 92. For a thorough assessment and comparison of studies that try to measure trends in prescription drug spending and utilization, see "Explaining the Growth in Prescription Drug Spending: A Review of Recent Studies," report prepared by Mark Merlis, Institute for Health Policy Solutions, for the U.S. Department of Health and Human Services, Conference on Pharmaceutical Pricing Practices, Utilization and Costs, Georgetown University, August 8–9, 2000, available at http://aspe.hhs.gov/health/reports/Drug-papers/merlis/Merlis-Final.htm.

28. Frank R. Lichtenberg, "Do (More and Better) Drugs Keep People out of Hospitals?" *American Economic Review* 86, no. 2 (May 1996): 384f.

29. Stephen B. Soumerai and Dennis Ross-Degnan, "Inadequate Prescription-Drug Coverage for Medicare Enrollees—A Call to Action," *New England Journal of Medicine* 340, no. 9 (March 4, 1999): 722–28.

30. *Budget Options,* Congressional Budget Office, February 2001, contains a good summary of the potential costs of a benefit under several designs embodied in bills introduced in the 107th Congress. See Chapter 2, "Expanding the Scope of Federal Retirement, Health, and Education Activities."

31. Christopher Hogan, Paul B. Ginsburg, and Jon R. Gabel, "Tracking Health Care Costs: Inflation Returns," *Health Affairs* 19, no. 6 (November/December 2000): 217–23.

32. Brian F. Gage et al., "Cost-Effectiveness of Warfarin and Aspirin for Prophylaxis of Stroke in Patients with Nonvalvular Atrial Fibrillation," *Journal of the American Medical Association* 274, no. 23. (December 20, 1995): 1839–45, cited in Kevin A. Schulman and Benjamin P. Linas,

"Pharmacoeconomics: State of the Art in 1997," *Annual Review of Public Health* 18 (1997): 529–48. See also Peter J. Neumann et al., "Are Pharmaceuticals Cost-Effective? A Review of the Evidence," *Health Affairs* 19, no. 2 (March/April 2000): 92–109.

33. Neumann et al., "Are Pharmaceuticals Cost-Effective?"

34. See, in particular, Peter D. Fox, "Prescription Drug Benefits: Cost Management Issues For Medicare," Public Policy Insitute, AARP, Washington, D.C., August 2000, available at http://research.aarp.org/health/2000_09_cost_1.html; Anna E. Cook, "Strategies for Containing Drug Costs: Implications for a Medicare Benefit," *Health Care Financing Review* 20, no. 3 (Spring 1999): 29–37.

35. Jacobzone, "Pharmaceutical Prices in OECD Countries," p. 23.

36. Thomas Burton, "Why Generic Drugs Often Can't Compete against Brand Names," *Wall Street Journal*, November 18, 1998, p. A1.

37. Nancy A. Whitelaw and Gail L. Warden, "Reexamining the Delivery System as Part of Medicare Reform," *Health Affairs* 18, no. 1 (January/February 1999): 132–43.

38. The effects of a Medicare prescription drug benefit, especially a universal benefit, on existing sources of coverage could be profound; the extent of this impact would depend heavily on the details of particular proposals. Most proposals try to take steps to avoid disrupting existing sources of drug coverage, especially employer-sponsored coverage. For instance, President Clinton's 1999 plan would have subsidized employers that offered retirees prescription coverage that was at least as generous as that proposed for the Medicare benefit.

39. For summaries and cost estimates of these plans, see especially "A Side-by-Side Comparison of Selected Medicare Prescription Drug Coverage Proposals," report prepared by Michael E. Gluck, Institute for Health Care Research Policy, for the Henry J. Kaiser Family Foundation, Washington, D.C., August 2000; letter from Dan Crippen, director, Congressional Budget Office, to Frank Lautenberg, U.S. Congress, Senate, Committee on the Budget, September 1, 2000, available at http://www.cbo.gov/showdoc.cfm?index=2378&sequence=0&from=7.

40. See, in particular, Stanley S. Wallack et al., "Sources of Growth in Pharmaceutical Expenditures," paper presented at the Seventh Princeton Conference, "Access to Pharmaceuticals," Woodrow Wilson School of Public Policy, Princeton University, May 11–13, 2000.

41. See statement of Chip Kahn, Health Insurance Association of America, quoted in Robert Pear, "House Approves a Medicare Prescription Benefit," *New York Times*, June 29, 2000, p. A1.

42. See "Low-Income Prescription Drug Plans: An Unworkable Prescription for America's Seniors," National Economic Council and Domestic Policy Council, September 18, 2000.

43. Fuchs et al., *Analyzing Options to Cover Prescription Drugs,* passim. Note that CBO director Dan Crippen, in his May 11, 2000, testimony, estimated that 7 percent spend more than $2000, not $4000. Stop-loss protections are included in both the Clinton and the Breaux-Frist plans. It is worth observing that under even the most generous drug benefit proposal, beneficiary premiums would be a significantly higher percentage of the cost of benefits received than for other services covered under Medicare.

44. "Medicare and Prescription Drugs," Henry J. Kaiser Family Foundation.

45. Christine K. Cassel, Richard W. Besdine, and Lydia C. Siegel, "Restructuring Medicare for the Next Century: What Will Beneficiaries Really Need?" *Health Affairs* 18, no. 1 (January/February 1999): 118–31.

46. Marilyn J. Field, Robert L. Lawrence, and Lee Zwanziger, eds., *Extending Medicare Coverage for Preventive and Other Services,* Institute of Medicine, Washington, D.C., 2000, pp. 13–25. Some 350 bills that attempted to add preventive services to Medicare were rejected before this one passed. Under standard insurance theory, smaller costs should be the responsibility of the policyholder (this is one rationale behind requiring deductibles), and larger costs should be borne by the insurer.

47. See, for example, John W. Rowe and Robert L. Kahn, *Successful Aging* (New York: Pantheon, 1998).

48. U.S. Department of Health and Human Services, Agency for Healthcare Research and Quality, *Guide to Clinical Preventive Services,* 2d ed., Report of the U.S. Preventive Services Task Force; U.S. Department of Health and Human Services, Public Health Service, "Healthy People: Progress Review—Cancer," April 7, 1998, point no. 16.13, available at http://odphp.osophs.dhhs.gov/pubs/hp2000/PROGRVW/Cancer/cancer.htm. Fecal occult blood tests are used to detect hidden blood in the stool.

49. Marian E. Gornick, *Vulnerable Populations and Medicare Services: Why Do Disparities Exist?* (New York: The Century Foundation Press, 2000), p. 30, Table 4.4.

50. See ibid., pp. 28–30 (Tables 4.2, 4.3 and 4.4); U.S. Department of Health and Human Services, *Guide to Clinical Preventive Services,* p. lxviii, Table 4.

51. P.L. 105-33, Sec. 4101–4108, August 5, 1997. See testimony of William Scanlon, director, Health Financing and Systems Issues, U.S. General Accounting Office, before the Special Committee on Aging, "Few Beneficiaries Use Colorectal Cancer Screening and Diagnostic Services," U.S. Congress, Senate, 106th Cong., 2d sess., March 6, 2000.

52. See "The President's Plan to Modernize and Strengthen Medicare for the 21st Century," National Economic Council and Domestic Policy Council, July 2, 1999, p. 27.

53. Robert Pear, "Clinton Raises Stakes in the Battle over a Bigger Medicare Pot," *New York Times,* November 1, 2000, p. A22.

54. Institute of Medicine, *The Role of Nutrition in Maintaining Health in the Nation's Elderly: Evaluating Coverage of Nutrition Services for the Medicare Population* (Washington, D.C.: National Academy Press, 2000); Field, Lawrence, and Zwanziger, *Extending Medicare Coverage for Preventive and Other Services.*

55. For background on this issue, see Mayur Desai et al., "Trends in Vision and Hearing Among Older Americans," *Aging Trends,* no. 2, National Center for Health Statistics, Centers for Disease Control and Prevention, Atlanta, March 2001, available at http://www.cdc.gov/nchs/data/agingtrends/02vision.pdf. Reimbursing the therapists who assist visually impaired seniors might be one initiative to consider in this area. See, for example, Judy Mann, "Bill Would Bring Needed Low-Vision Therapy," *Washington Post,* July 19, 2000, p. C13.

CHAPTER 4

1. See Bruce Vladeck and Kathleen King, "Medicare at 30: Preparing for the Future," *Journal of the American Medical* Association 274, no. 3 (July 19, 1995): 259.

2. Within Medicare, vulnerable populations are understood to be "beneficiaries with characteristics or circumstances that may hinder access to appropriate health services," with access understood as the "timely, adequate, and necessary delivery of health care." Medicare Payment Advisory Commission, *Report to the Congress: Context for a Changing Medicare Program,* June 1998, p. 143.

3. See, in particular, Madonna Harrington Meyer, "Gender, Generations, and Chronic Conditions," *Public Policy and Aging Report* 11, no. 2 (Winter 2001), National Academy on an Aging Society, Washington, D.C., pp. 1, 7–10.

4. As of 1996, 83 percent of beneficiaries were white, while 9 percent were African-American and 6 percent of Hispanic background. Less than 2 percent of beneficiaries had another ethnic background, such as Asian-American. The number of minority beneficiaries, and especially Latino beneficiaries, is expected to rise substantially in the future. Health Care Financing Administration, *A Profile of Medicare: Chart Book,* May 1998, Figure 6.

5. Marian E. Gornick, *Vulnerable Populations and Medicare Services: Why Do Disparities Exist?* (New York: The Century Foundation, 2000), pp. 25–35.

6. "Medicare's Role for Latinos," fact sheet, Henry J. Kaiser Family Foundation, Washington, D.C., April 1999; "Background on the Impact of Health Care Proposals for Quality Health Care and Prescription Drug Coverage," Office of the Press Secretary, The White House, July 28, 1999.

7. Health Care Financing Administration, Medicare Current Beneficiary Survey, 1997, Table 1.6, "Demographic and Socioeconomic Characteristics of Nonistitutionalized Medicare Beneficiaries, by Insurance Coverage, 1997."

8. Karen Scott Collins, et al., *U.S. Minority Health: A Chart Book*, Commonwealth Fund, New York, 1999, Chart 5.5.

9. Carol J. R. Hogue, Martha A. Hargraves, and Karen Scott Collins ed., *Minority Health in America: Findings and Policy Implications from the Commonwealth Fund Minority Health Survey* (Baltimore: Johns Hopkins University Press, 2000), p. xiii.

10. See James A. Auerbach, Barbara Kivimae Krimgold, and Bonnie Lefkowitz, *Improving Health: It Doesn't Take a Revolution* (Washington, D.C.: National Policy Association and Academy for Health Services Research and Health Policy, 2000), p. 7.

11. Though these discrepancies are better documented than understood, researchers have identified a number of plausible contributing causes: cultural issues (such as higher stress) and behavioral traits (such as diet), biological differences (African-Americans appear more prone than whites to contract chronic illnesses such as diabetes), and the structure of the medical profession, including the possibility of racial discrimination on the part of some providers.

12. "Do Young Retirees and Older Workers Differ by Race?" *Data Profiles: Young Retirees and Older Workers*, no. 4, National Academy on an Aging Society, Washington, D.C., December 2000.

13. Margo L. Rosenbach and JoAnn Lamphere, "Bridging the Gaps between Medicare and Medicaid: The Case of QMBs and SLMBs," paper no. 9902, Public Policy Institute, AARP, Washington, D.C., January 1999, p. 1, available at http://research.aarp.org/health/9902_qmbs.html.

14. "Shortchanged: Billions Withheld from Medicare Beneficiaries," Families USA, Washington, D.C., July 1998. See also Marilyn Moon, Niall Brennan, and Misha Segal, "Improving Coverage for Low-Income Medicare Beneficiaries," Commonwealth Fund, New York, December 1998.

15. Marsha Gold and Natalie Justh, "Forced Exit: Beneficiaries in Plans Terminating in 2000," *Monitoring Medicare+Choice: Fast Facts*, no. 3, Mathematica Policy Research, Princeton, N.J., September 2000; "Medicare HMOs Serve Many Financially Vulnerable Beneficiaries," *Facts & Figures*, American Association of Health Plans, Washington, D.C., May 17, 2000.

16. "Medicare and Women: The Faces of Medicare," Henry J. Kaiser Family Foundation, Washington, D.C., 2000; Mary J. Gibson and Normandy Brangan, "Out-of-Pocket Spending on Health Care by Women Age 65 and Over in Fee-for-Service Medicare: 1998 Projections" Public Policy Institute, AARP, Washington, D.C., November 1998, available at http://research.aarp.org/health/fs72_oldwm.html.

17. Stephanie Maxwell, Marilyn Moon, and Misha Segal, "Growth in Medicare and Out-of-Pocket Spending: Impact on Vulnerable Beneficiaries," Commonwealth Fund, New York, January 2001.

18. U.S. Department of Health and Human Services, *Report to the President: Prescription Drug Coverage, Spending, Utilization, and Prices*, April 2000, p. 78, available at http://aspe.hhs.gov/health/reports/drugstudy/.

19. One study, in fact, suggests that financial risk and health outcomes may be correlated in some instances; its authors found that Medicare beneficiaries with private supplemental coverage who were better protected from the risk of high out-of-pocket expenses lived longer than those who had less generous supplemental coverage. See Mark P. Doescher et al., "Supplemental Insurance and Mortality in Elderly Americans: Findings from a National Cohort," *Archives of Family Medicine* 9, no. 3 (March 2000): 251–57.

20. Many experts have hoped that managed care plans, because they contribute to the vertical integration of health systems and offer incentives for prevention, would contribute to the coordination of care for their members. Others feared that fixed per person payments would encourage plans not to treat the disabled and those with serious health problems. The evidence is mixed. Few if any studies have shown that managed care plans to date have helped frailer and sicker patients, and some have argued that disabled patients fare slightly worse in managed care. Medicare also pays for several small-scale managed care programs that serve frail beneficiaries by combining elements of acute and long-term care, usually with the aim of helping patients stay at home and reducing the incidence of hospitalization. The most important of these programs are the Program of All-Inclusive Care for the Elderly (PACE), now a permanent option within Medicare, and social health maintenance organizations (SHMOs). Because these programs are extremely small and localized, it is hard to generalize from their experience.

21. In a report submitted to HCFA on the potential of coordinated care programs, researchers from Mathematica Policy Research intensively studied twenty-nine programs in a search for "best practices" in this area. Based on this study of mostly disease management and case management strategies, they concluded that "our study suggests that incremental approaches to improving chronic illness can succeed." Arnold Chen et al., *Best Practices in Coordinated Care*, Mathematica Policy Research, Princeton, N.J., March 22, 2000.

22. See "Chronic Conditions: A Challenge for the 21st Century," *Data Profiles: Chronic and Disabling Conditions*, no. 1, National Academy on an Aging Society, Washington, D.C., November 1999. According to estimates made by the Robert Wood Johnson Foundation, the number of persons with chronic conditions is expected to reach 148 million by the year 2030.

23. Christine K. Cassel, Richard W. Besdine, and Lydia C. Siegel, "Restructuring Medicare for the Next Century: What Will Beneficiaries Really Need?" *Health Affairs* 18, no. 1 (January/ February 1999): 118–31; "The Aging Factor in Health and Disease: The Promise of Basic Research on Aging," International Longevity Center-USA, Mount Sinai School of

Medicine, February 1999. In 2000, HCFA began offering a health care scholarship for geriatricians, but it funds just a single recipient each year.

24. Medicare pays for skilled nursing care when a physician certifies that an episode of acute care for a patient has occurred and for a limited number of home health visits following hospitalization. Because the program does not cover long-term care per se, it funds a much smaller percentage of nursing home care than Medicaid, the joint federal-state program for those who have very limited resources and who satisfy other demographic eligibility criteria.

25. Nancy A. Whitelaw and Gail L. Warden, "Reexamining the Delivery System as Part of Medicare Reform," *Health Affairs* 18, no. 1 (January/February 1999): 137.

26. Cassel, Besdine, and Siegel, "Restructuring Medicare for the Next Century."

27. Carol Cronin, "Reaching and Educating Medicare Beneficiaries About Choice," in Institute of Medicine, Choice and Managed Care Committee, *Improving the Medicare Market: Adding Choice and Protections* (Washington, D.C.: National Academy Press, 1996), pp. 236–69.

28. Medicare Payment Advisory Commission, *Report to the Congress: Medicare in Rural America*, June 2001, passim. This report looks comprehensively and in great detail at the issues facing Medicare and its rural beneficiaries.

29. Lisa H. Green et al., *Medicare State Profiles: State and Regional Data on Medicare and the Population It Serves*, Henry J. Kaiser Family Foundation, Washington, D.C., September 1999.

30. Ibid.

31. Jonathan Skinner, "Medicare Reform: Improving Fairness and Efficiency," Center for the Evaluative Clinical Sciences, Dartmouth Medical School, n.d., available at http://www.dartmouthatlas.org/medicarereform/medicare_reform.php.

32. "A Rural Assessment of Leading Proposals to Redesign the Medicare Program," Rural Policy Research Institute, University of Missouri, May 31, 2000, p. 1.

33. Medicare Payment Advisory Commission, *Report to Congress: Medicare in Rural America*, pp. 115–23.

34. See "A Rural Assessment of Leading Proposals to Redesign the Medicare Program," pp. 17–19, for a broader discussion of possible policy alternatives.

CHAPTER 5

1. Bruce Vladeck, "The Political Economy of Medicare," *Health Affairs* 18, no. 1 (January/February 1999): 27. This article by Vladeck, the former administrator of HCFA, is a good short introduction to Medicare's impact on the health industry and the political realities of the program.

2. See Center for the Evaluative Clinical Sciences, Dartmouth Medical School, *The Dartmouth Atlas of Health Care in the United States* (Chicago: American Hospital Publishing, Inc., 1998).

3. Linda T. Kohn, *To Err is Human: Building a Safer Health System* (Washington, D.C.: National Academy Press, 2000).

4. President's Advisory Commission on Consumer Protection and Quality in the Health Care Industry, *Quality First: Better Health Care for All Americans*, March 1998, Chapter 1, available at http://www.hcqualitycommission.gov/.

5. Health economist David Dranove describes these issues as the characteristic "shopping problem" of health care, noting that "it is difficult for any person or any organization, be they patient, physician, managed care organization, or the government, to be an efficient and effective purchaser of health care goods and services." Dranove's book, *The Economic Evolution of American Health Care: From Marcus Welby to Managed Care* (Princeton, N.J.: Princeton University Press, 2000), is a highly accessible summary of changes in the health care delivery system since the 1960s.

6. Ibid., p. 24.

7. On the definitions of quality, see Mark A. Schuster, Elizabeth A. McGlynn, and Robert H. Brook, "How Good is the Quality of Health Care in the United States?" *Milbank Quarterly* 76, no. 4 (December 1998): 517–63; Paul Starr, "Health Care Reform and the New Economy," *Health Affairs* 19, no. 6 (November/December 2000): 27–28. For an overview of a "CQI" approach to health delivery, see Mark R. Chassin, "Is Health Care Ready for Six Sigma Quality?" *Milbank Quarterly* 76, no. 4 (December 1998): 565–92.

8. On this point, see the history of medicine by Roy Porter, *The Greatest Benefit to Mankind: A Medical History of Humanity* (New York: W. W. Norton and Co., 1998).

9. On this issue, see Michael L. Millenson, *Demanding Medical Excellence: Doctors and Accountability in the Information Age* (Chicago: University of Chicago Press, 1997), passim.

10. See, on this point, James C. Robinson, *The Corporate Practice of Medicine: Competition and Innovation in Health Care* (Berkeley.: University of California Press, 1999).

11. Milton I. Roemer and Max Schoen, "Hospital Utilization under Insurance," Monograph no. 6, American Hospital Association, Chicago, 1959; summary in *Hospitals*, September 16, 1959, pp. 36–37.

12. Center for the Evaluative Clinical Sciences, *Dartmouth Atlas of Health Care.*

13. Stephen B. Soumerai et al., "Adverse Outcomes of Underuse of Beta-Blockers in Elderly Survivors of Acute Myocardial Infarction, *Journal of the American Medical Association* 277 (January 8, 1997): 115–21.

14. Quoted in Millenson, *Demanding Medical Excellence*, p. 48.

15. Institute of Medicine, *Crossing the Quality Chasm: A New Health System for the 21st Century* (Washington, D.C.: National Academy Press, 2001), Chapter 7.

16. This "triadic" schema of quality measurement was developed by the late Avedis Donabedian. See Dranove, *Economic Evaluation of American Health Care,* p. 144; and Fitzhugh Mullan, "A Founder of Quality Assessment Encounters a Troubled System Firsthand," *Health Affairs* 20, no. 1 (January/February 2001): 137–41.

17. Dranove, *Economic Evaluation of American Health Care,* p. 145.

18. See David M. Eddy, "Perfomance Measurement: Problems and Solutions," *Health Affairs* 17, no. 4 (July/August 1998): 7–25.

19. Starr, "Health Care Reform and the New Economy," pp. 23–32.

20. See Eddy, "Performance Measurement."

21. Dranove, *Economic Evaluation of American Health Care,* pp. 57–58.

22. Ibid.

23. As researchers from the Lewin Group, a major health care consulting firm, put it, "the state of the art in quality assurance has shifted to the continuous quality improvement (CQI) model, which de-emphasizes structural indicators and identification of instances of quality deficiencies while focusing on a continuous process of measuring outcomes and development of initiatives to improve performance." John F. Sheils et al., "Quality Health Care: New Challenges as Medicare Evolves," Medicare Series Report prepared by the Lewin Group for the National Coalition on Health Care, Washington, D.C., January 26, 1999; see Millenson, *Demanding Medical Excellence,* p. 257; Stephen M. Shortell, Charles L. Bennett, and Gayle R. Byck, "Assessing the Impact of Continuous Quality Improvement on Clinical Practice: What It Will Take to Accelerate Progress," *Milbank Quarterly* 76, no. 4 (December 1998): 593–624. Reflecting this new mission, members of peer review organizations now generally prefer their groups to be referred to as QIOs, or quality improvement organizations. See "The Role of the PROs," Issue Brief, vol. 2, no. 2, Center for Medicare Education, Institute for the Future of Aging Services, Washington, D.C., 2001.

24. Medicare Payment Advisory Commission, *Report to the Congress: Selected Medicare Issues,* June 1999, p. 22. Extensive antifraud legislation also has had significant effects.

25. Ibid., p. 28.

26. Sheils et al., "Quality Health Care," p. 27.

27. Medicare Payment Advisory Commission, *Report to the Congress: Selected Medicare Issues,* June 2000, p. 96.

28. See, in particular, Allan Baumgarten, "Case Studies in Reducing Regulatory Duplication in Managed Care," report prepared for the California HealthCare Foundation, Oakland, August 2000.

29. Eddy, "Performance Measurement," p. 16.

30. Stephen F. Jencks et al., "Quality of Medical Care Delivered to Medicare Beneficiaries: A Profile at State and National Levels," *Journal of the American Medical Association* 284, no. 13 (October 4, 2000): 1670–76.

31. *The State of Managed Care Quality 1999,* National Committee for Quality Assurance, Washington, D.C., 1999.

32. *From a Generation Behind to a Generation Ahead: Transforming Traditional Medicare,* Final Report of the Study Panel on Fee-for-Service Medicare, National Academy of Social Insurance, Washington, D.C., January 1998. This report offers a fuller and more detailed description of these strategies.

33. "The President's Plan to Modernize and Strengthen Medicare for the 21st Century," National Economic Council and Domestic Policy Council, July 2, 1999.

34. See the issue brief authored by the Foundation for Accountability, "Health Care Choices: Sharing the Quality Message," Issue Brief, vol. 2, no. 1, Center for Medicare Education, Institute for the Future of Aging Services, Washington, D.C., 2001; see also the Leapfrog Group website, available at http://leapfroggroup.org.

35. See Irene Fraser et al., "The Pursuit of Quality by Business Coalitions: A National Survey," *Health Affairs* 18, no. 6 (November/December 1999): 158–65.

36. Such value-purchasing efforts also are supported by consortia that have launched important initiatives designed to measure and promote high-quality health care. The Alliance of Community Health Plans, for example, has devised its Benchmarks in Quality in Safety to promote improvements in the overall health of a target population; an initiative called RxMedicine, sponsored by a number of organizations including Blue Cross and Blue Shield, is attempting to assess the relative value of new-to-the-market pre-scription drugs.

37. See *From a Generation Behind to a Generation Ahead: Transforming Traditional Medicare,* p. 27f.

CHAPTER 6

1. See Stanley B. Jones and Marion Ein Lewin, eds., *Improving the Medicare Market: Adding Choice and Protections* (Washington, D.C.: National Academy Press, 1996).

2. These are essentially HMOs organized by provider groups rather than by insurance companies.

3. The first private fee-for-service plan has been approved by HCFA as an offering in the year 2001. The product is now available in some entire states and in parts of other states across the country. As of March, 2001, nearly 11,500 people on Medicare had enrolled in this plan across the country.

4. Lauren MacCormack et al., "Health Insurance Knowledge among Medicare Beneficiaries," Health Care Financing Administration and Agency for Healthcare Research and Quality, 2000.

5. Judith H. Hibbard et al., "Can Medicare Beneficiaries Make Informed Choices?" *Health Affairs* 17, no. 6 (November/December 1998): 181–93.

6. George Loewenstein, "Is More Choice Always Better?" Social Security Brief no. 7, National Academy of Social Insurance, Washington, D.C., October 1999.

7. Much of the relevant research is summarized in Jones and Lewin, *Improving the Medicare Market.* Specific studies in this area include "Analysis of Focus Groups Concerning Managed Care and Medicare," report prepared by Frederick/Schneiders Inc. for the Henry J. Kaiser Family Foundation, Washington, D.C., March 1995; Susan Edgman-Levitan and Paul D. Cleary, "What Information Do Consumers Want and Need? *Health Affairs* 15, no. 4 (Winter 1996): 42–56; and Shoshanna Sofaer and M. Margo Hurwicz, "When Medical Group and HMO Part Company: Disenrollment Decisions in Medicare HMO's," *Medical Care* 31 (1993): 808–21. Focus group and case study evidence indicates that consumer response to Medicare HMOs is quite different in the more mature managed care markets, where HMOs in general as well as Medicare HMOs have been a part of the landscape for many more years. In these markets, consumers are more aware of and interested in quality differences among available HMOs and are often more concerned about the breadth and quality of the provider network as a whole rather than the availability of one or more specific doctors or other providers. Indeed, they value having a well-screened list of providers to choose from.

8. National Adult Literacy Survey, National Center for Education Statistics, Washington, D.C., 1992.

9. Nelda McCall, Thomas Rice, and Judith Sangl, "Consumer Knowledge of Medicare and Supplemental Health Insurance Benefits," *Health Services Research* 20 (February 1986): 633–57.

10. This task will become more pressing when (and if) a single annual enrollment period comes to pass, as now scheduled, in the fall of 2003 for the year 2004.

11. See Marsha Gold et al., "Medicare Beneficiaries and Health Plan Choice, 2000," *Monitoring Medicare+Choice,* Mathematica Policy Research, Princeton, N.J., January 2001.

12. Institute of Medicine, *Crossing the Quality Chasm: A New Health System for the 21st Century* (Washington, D.C.: National Academy Press, 2001). See especially Chapter 7, "Using Information Technology."

13. See Beth Stevens and Jessica Mittler, "Making Medicare+Choice Real: Understanding and Meeting the Information Needs of Beneficiaries at the Local Level," *Monitoring Medicare+Choice,* Mathematica Policy Research, Princeton, N.J., November 2000.

CHAPTER 7

1. One task force member suggested a possible way for improving the adequacy of Medicare's administrative budget over time. This would involve setting it through an appropriation from the trust fund, perhaps as a fixed percentage of benefits paid, rather than through the current practice of appropriations through the Department of Health and Human Services budget as a whole. (The administrative budget for Social Security and for peer review organizations within Medicare are currently set through trust fund appropriations.) This change might relieve Medicare administrators from having to compete for their budgetary needs with other departments within HHS.

2. See testimony of Richard F. Corlin, president-elect, American Medical Association, before the Subcommittee on Health, "Medicare Reform: Bringing Regulatory Relief to Beneficiaries and Providers," U.S. Congress, House, Committee on Ways and Means, 107th Cong., 1st sess., March 15, 2001. The transcripts from these hearings, which represent an excellent set of perspectives on administrative and operational issues within Medicare, may be accessed at http://waysandmeans.house.gov/health/107cong/hl-2wit.htm.

3. "Crisis Facing HCFA & Millions of Americans," open letter to Congress and the executive, *Health Affairs* 18, no. 1 (January/February 1999): 8–10.

4. See Lynn Etheredge, "Medicare and Regulations," from unpublished conference presentation, "Medicare: The Crisis in Governance," The Heritage Foundation, Washington D.C., June 12, 2001.

5. For example, the Medicare Payment Advisory Commission described the regulations proposed for enacting a Minimum Data Set for Post-Acute Care—a measure it supported in principle—as "notably lengthy and complex." This evaluation tool, designed to collect data for assessing the appropriateness of Medicare payments and for monitoring quality, includes more than four hundred items and seven different time frames under which a patient's condition must be assessed. Medicare Payment Advisory Commission, *Report to the Congress: Medicare Payment Policy*, March 2001, p. 93.

6. See Bruce C. Vladeck and Barbara S. Cooper, "Making Medicare Work Better," Institute for Medicare Practice, Mount Sinai School of Medicine, March 2001, available at http://www.mssm.edu/instituteformedicare/pdfs/FINALFIL.PDF; Corlin, "Medicare Reform: Bringing Regulatory Relief."

7. Most comprehensive Medicare reform proposals—including President Clinton's 1999 proposal and the Breaux-Frist premium support plan of the same year—have contained provisions aimed at the administrative modernization of the program. The former proposed that more flexibility in hiring personnel be granted and urged the creation of oversight panels to

recommend new coverage of benefits, better customer relations, and purchasing innovations. (See "The President's Plan to Modernize and Strengthen Medicare for the 21st Century," National Economic Council and Domestic Policy Council, July 2, 1999, pp. 18–19.) The latter proposed the idea of a new Medicare Board that would replace HCFA, overseeing a restructured Medicare program based on competition among plans. ("Medicare Preservation and Improvement Act of 1999," S.1895, 106th Cong., 1st sess.)

8. For in-depth analysis of the many proposals and issues for changes to the administration of Medicare, see David Walker, "Major Management Challenges and Program Risks," GAO/OCG-99-7, U.S. General Accounting Office, January 1999; William J. Scanlon, "Medicare: 21st Century Challenges Prompt Fresh Thinking about Program's Administrative Structure," GAO/T-HEHS-00-108, U.S. General Accounting Office, May 4, 2000; "Medicare Governance: The Health Care Financing Administration's Role and Readiness in Reform," hearing before the Committee on Finance, U.S. Congress, Senate, 106th Cong., 2d sess., May 4, 2000, available at http://www.senate.gov/~finance/w5-4-0.htm; Lynn Etheredge, "Medicare's Governance and Structure: A Proposal," *Health Affairs* 19, no. 5 (September/October 2000): 60–71.

COMPETITION-BASED APPROACHES TO MEDICARE REFORM

LISA POTETZ

ACKNOWLEDGMENTS

The author is grateful for the support of The Century Foundation and The Commonwealth Fund and for the efforts of Greg Anrig, Brian Biles, and Susan Raetzman in initiating and overseeing the project. Leif Wellington Haase provided thoughtful comments and advice throughout.

This paper largely summarizes the work of many health and Medicare policy experts. The author is indebted to those who took the time to review earlier drafts, including Beth Fuchs, Julie James, Marilyn Moon, Patricia Neuman, Shoshanna Sofaer, and Marina Weiss. Their comments were invaluable, but any deficiencies in the final product are the sole responsibility of the author.

1

WHY REFORM MEDICARE?

Despite Medicare's standing as one of the most popular and successful government programs, policymakers are in the early stages of an important, and probably lengthy, debate about its future shape. Over the past thirty-five years, the federal government has maintained a commitment to pay for health care services provided to elderly and disabled Americans. (See "A Medicare Overview," page 130.) The debate over Medicare reform is focused on how to continue that obligation into the twenty-first century.

The popularity of Medicare is well merited, given its success. It is easy now to take for granted this program of universal health insurance coverage for the elderly, but prior to the enactment of Medicare in 1965, almost half of elderly Americans had no health insurance coverage.[1] Since its inception, Medicare has improved access to health care services, helped protect its beneficiaries against the financial burdens of medical costs, and contributed to the improved aggregate health status of the elderly.[2] Polls show Medicare to be a valued, if not always well understood, program.[3] Some 77 percent of Americans of all ages say it is "very important" to them that the Medicare program be preserved for future retirees.[4]

Concern about both the long-term sustainability of Medicare financing and the need for improvements in program benefits are fueling the debate over Medicare reform.

A MEDICARE OVERVIEW

Who Is Covered?	Some 39 million Americans are enrolled in Medicare, including 34 million elderly and 5 million disabled persons. Most individuals become eligible for Medicare at age sixty-five. Individuals receiving Social Security disability benefits or with permanent kidney failure also are eligible for coverage.
Covered Services	Part A (Hospital Insurance) covers inpatient hospital stays, up to one hundred days of skilled nursing facility (SNF) care following a hospital stay, home health visits following a hospital or SNF stay, and hospice care. Part B (Supplementary Medical Insurance) covers physician and outpatient hospital visits, home health care not covered under Part A, X-rays, laboratory services, certain cancer screenings and other preventive benefits, physical therapy, occupational therapy, speech therapy, and durable medical equipment.
Beneficiary Cost Sharing	The inpatient hospital deductible was $776 in 2000, with cost sharing of $194 for days 61–90 and $388 for days 91–150; SNF cost sharing was $97 for days 21–100. The annual Part B deductible was $100 and 20 percent cost sharing was required for most Part B services.
Expenditures	$211 billion was spent in fiscal year 1999; $129 billion (61 percent) for Part A benefits, $79 billion (37 percent) for Part B benefits, and $3 billion (less than 2 percent) for program administration.
Sources of Financing	Part A is financed by a payroll tax of 2.9 percent (1.45 percent employer/1.45 percent employee). Payroll taxes are deposited into the Hospital Insurance Trust Fund for the sole purpose of paying for Part A benefits. Part B is financed by a combination of beneficiary premiums (25 percent) and general revenue (75 percent). The Part B premium for 2000 was $45.50 a month; it is projected to increase to $85.90 a month by 2009.
Role of Managed Care	More than 6 million beneficiaries (16 percent) are enrolled in health maintenance organizations and other managed care plans for their Medicare benefits.

Sources: Medicare Enrollment Trends, 1966–1998, Health Care Financing Administration, U.S. Department of Health and Human Services, June 30, 1999; *Your Medicare Benefits,* Health Care Financing Administration, U.S. Department of Health and Human Services, 1999; *Medicare Deductible, Coinsurance and Premium Amounts for 2000,* Health Care Financing Administration, U.S. Department of Health and Human Services, October 25, 1999; *Monthly Report: Medicare Managed Care Plans,* Health Care Financing Administration, U.S. Department of Health and Human Services, July 2000; *2000 Annual Report of the Board of Trustees of the Supplementary Medical Insurance Trust Fund,* Health Care Financing Administration, U.S. Department of Health and Human Services, March 30, 2000, p. 64.

GUARANTEEING FUTURE FINANCING

Medicare's financing problem is driven by the demographic shifts associated with the aging of the baby-boom generation into Medicare eligibility, beginning in 2011. The existing structure of program financing through a combination of payroll taxes, beneficiary premiums, and general revenue will be severely strained as the number of workers per enrollee falls from 4.0 in 1999 to 2.3 by 2030—the point at which the last of the baby boomers will just be gaining Medicare eligibility.[5] In particular, the Hospital Insurance Trust Fund, which currently finances about 60 percent of Medicare expenditures, is expected to begin to draw down its reserve funds in 2017 and to become completely insolvent in the year 2025.[6]

In addition to the demographic pressures, economywide trends in health care inflation contribute to Medicare's financing problems. Over time, national spending on health care services has grown faster than general inflation, and health care has risen as a share of the economy—from 5.7 percent of the gross domestic product in 1965 to 13.5 percent in 1998.[7] Similarly, since its inception, Medicare spending per enrollee has grown an average of three to four percentage points more than inflation each year.[8] This trend helped make Medicare a favored target of budget cutters during the 1980s and 1990s as concern about soaring federal deficits grew. In addition to being one of the largest federal programs, Medicare attracted budget cutters' attention because its complexity permitted the use of a variety of policy levers to generate the program savings needed to meet deficit reduction goals.

Recently, the short-term financial picture for Medicare has improved significantly. Medicare spending actually fell by about $1.7 billion in fiscal year 1999, and the trend line indicating slower spending growth continues.[9] This contrasts with recent trends in private health insurance. After several years of historically low growth (averaging 3.2 percent a year for 1995–97), private health insurance expenditures rose by 8.2 percent in 1998.[10] The Congressional Budget Office has attributed the downturn in the rate of Medicare spending to relatively slow growth in enrollment, antifraud initiatives designed to eliminate unnecessary program spending, and specific cost-containment provisions of the Balanced Budget Act of 1997 (Pub. Law 105-33).[11] Despite this apparent turnaround, an ongoing struggle against rising health care costs is anticipated for both Medicare and private health insurance plans as both the volume and cost of medical services continue to increase.

IMPROVEMENTS IN MEDICARE BENEFITS

In addition to the obvious concerns about long-term program financing, the structure of Medicare benefits is a target of reform as
well. At the time of its enactment, Medicare was designed to resemble a typical private health insurance plan, guaranteeing coverage
for inpatient hospital stays and offering optional coverage for physician visits and other outpatient services. As standard insurance benefits have evolved since 1965, Medicare benefits have not kept pace,
and the program lacks the scope of coverage taken for granted by
most Americans with employer-based health insurance. In fact,
Medicare benefits on average cover only about half the health care
costs of the elderly.[12]

In particular, the Medicare program does not cover outpatient
prescription drugs and has no cap on the amount a beneficiary might
pay in deductibles and copayments. Growing recognition of the burden of prescription drug costs for the elderly made drug coverage the
focus of considerable debate in the 106th Congress. Despite the
prevalence of prescription drug benefits purchased through
"Medigap" policies and employer-sponsored supplemental insurance,
about 30 percent of beneficiaries have no prescription drug coverage.[13] More broadly, the average Medicare beneficiary spent about 19
percent of his or her income in 1998 on out-of-pocket costs for
Medicare cost sharing and acute health care needs not fully covered
by the program, a proportion projected to increase to 25 percent by
2025.[14] Finally, as an acute care health program, Medicare does not
serve the long-term care needs of the elderly and disabled. To date,
proposals for Medicare reform have not addressed the issue of long-
term care.

Because of these gaps in the benefit package, supplemental coverage is important to Medicare beneficiaries, a fact that needs to be
taken into account in considering the effects of various proposals
for Medicare reform. In 1996, only about 9 percent of Medicare beneficiaries lacked supplemental coverage of any kind. About 35 percent had retiree health benefits; 26 percent purchased individual
Medigap policies; 12 percent received Medicaid assistance for low-
income Medicare beneficiaries; and 9 percent had supplementary
benefits through Medicare managed care plans. The remaining 9
percent of beneficiaries switched among these categories during the
year.[15] Since 1996, enrollment in Medicare managed care plans has

increased—about 16 percent of beneficiaries were enrolled in such plans in July 2000.[16] Individual Medigap coverage can be expensive, often making a less expensive managed care option attractive to beneficiaries in those areas where it is available. For example, Medicare supplemental (Medigap) Plan C (which covers all deductibles and coinsurance but not prescription drugs and is the most popular of the ten standardized plan options) ranges in price for a sixty-five-year-old in 2000 from about $1700 to $2200 in Miami and from roughly $900 to $1700 in Cleveland.[17] In contrast, beneficiaries may, for no additional premium, be able to enroll in a managed care plan that eliminates the Medicare deductibles and limits copayments to only $5 or $10 per visit.

Medicaid provides important assistance to some low-income beneficiaries, but gaps in coverage remain. Furthermore, low-income individuals often have greater health care needs. Some very low-income beneficiaries qualify for full Medicaid benefits that wrap around Medicare, including prescription drug coverage and long-term care, as well as coverage of Medicare premiums and cost sharing. (See "Overview of Medicaid Assistance for Low-Income Medicare Beneficiaries," page 134.) Other beneficiaries are eligible for Medicaid payment of their cost sharing or the Part B premium, or both, but many who are eligible for these programs do not participate because they are not aware of them or because enrollment procedures are complex. Less than half of beneficiaries with incomes below the poverty line have any Medicaid coverage to supplement Medicare.[18] Coordination between Medicare and Medicaid coverage for these individuals is often complicated by differences between Medicaid and Medicare managed care programs. For example, some states require them to enroll in a Medicaid managed care plan, effectively eliminating choices of plans and health care providers generally available to Medicare beneficiaries.[19]

Lower-income beneficiaries who do not qualify for Medicaid or who are eligible but are not receiving Medicaid assistance may not be able to afford an individual Medigap policy. Some lower-income individuals have been able to obtain supplemental benefits by enrolling in Medicare managed care plans, which often provide additional coverage for little or no cost beyond the Part B premium.

Medicare's benefit structure and the complexities of supplemental coverage weigh significantly in the debate over Medicare reform. While the main motivation for reform may be concern about

OVERVIEW OF MEDICAID ASSISTANCE FOR
LOW-INCOME MEDICARE BENEFICIARIES

Full Medicaid Coverage	Supplemental Security Income recipients and certain other individuals may receive full Medicaid benefits to wrap around Medicare, including prescription drugs, long-term care, and coverage of Medicare cost sharing.
Qualified Medicare Beneficiary (QMB)	Individuals with incomes below 100 percent of the poverty level ($8,350 for an individual in 2000) who are not eligible for full Medicaid coverage may receive Medicaid coverage for the Part B premium. Medicare cost sharing is covered as well, but states are not required to pay cost sharing if the Medicaid payment rate is lower.
Specified Low-Income Beneficiary (SLMB)	Individuals with incomes between 100 and 120 percent of the poverty level are eligible for coverage of the Part B premium.
Qualifying Individuals	Federal block grants to states are issued through 2002 to provide Part B premium assistance to individuals with incomes between 120 percent and 175 percent of the poverty level who also meet an assets test. Federal funding is capped, and individuals are assisted on a first-come, first-served basis. Those with incomes between 120 percent and 135 percent of the poverty level may receive a full Part B premium subsidy; those between 135 percent and 175 percent may receive a partial subsidy.

Source: Andy Schneider, Kristen Fennel, and Patricia Keenan, *Medicaid Eligibility and the Elderly* (Washington, D.C.: Kaiser Commission on Medicaid and the Uninsured, May 1999), pp. 10–22.

how to ensure program financing for the long term, in considering the effect on beneficiaries, reform proposals must take into account the gaps in Medicare benefits and existing patterns of supplemental coverage.

FOCUSING THE DEBATE: THE MEDICARE COMMISSION

The National Bipartisan Commission on the Future of Medicare was created under the Balanced Budget Act of 1997 for the purpose of developing recommendations to Congress and the president on how to solve the long-term financing challenges facing the Medicare program. The commission was composed of seventeen members appointed jointly by President Clinton and the bipartisan congressional leadership and was cochaired by Senator John Breaux (D-La.) and Representative Bill Thomas (R-Calif.). The commission was required to report those recommendations that achieved the support of at least eleven of its seventeen members.

While the commission just failed to meet that supermajority requirement and did not submit a formal final report, its deliberations helped identify critical issues in the debate over Medicare reform. In particular, the proposal for a "premium support" approach to Medicare reform authored by the commission's cochairs and debated by the commission as a whole has formed the basis of one of the two major, competing legislative initiatives for Medicare reform.

The rest of this paper addresses the central question growing out of the National Bipartisan Commission's deliberations: To what extent should the Medicare program rely on competition among private health insurance plans to provide benefits to its enrollees? Chapter 2 discusses general approaches to Medicare reform, focusing on the theoretical underpinnings of plan competition and the premium support model and briefly describing competition mechanisms currently in place in the health benefits plan for federal employees and in Medicare. In Chapter 3, specific proposals for increasing plan competition in Medicare are examined. In particular, proposed legislation advancing the premium support model is contrasted with President Clinton's approach to Medicare reform.

2

MEDICARE REFORM AND COMPETITION AMONG HEALTH PLANS

Reforms to Medicare suggested in recent years range from relatively small, incremental steps to a more sweeping reconfiguration of the program. The proposals vary in their comprehensiveness, in the complexity of the program restructuring they would require, and, most important, in their potential effect on the ways in which current and future Medicare beneficiaries will obtain and pay for health care services.

Increasing the Medicare program's reliance on competition among private health plans is an element common to the two major, competing legislative proposals for Medicare reform, which will be discussed in Chapter 3. The degree and manner of the proposed reliance on private plans also is the major distinction between the two approaches.

In order best to understand these issues, this chapter outlines several approaches to health plan competition that have helped to shape the current debate. These are the theoretical approaches known as "managed competition" and "defined contribution" and the existing models of plan competition found in the Federal Employees Health Benefits Program and in Medicare+Choice (see "Competition and Medicare," page 138).

MANAGED COMPETITION AS THE BASIS FOR REFORM

Many proposals for health financing reform, both systemwide and Medicare-specific, rely in some fashion on the managed competition concept initially described by Alain Enthoven and others.[1] For

COMPETITION AND MEDICARE: A GLOSSARY OF TERMS

Defined Benefit	Individuals are entitled to benefits defined as coverage for specific health care services. Benefits are not tied to the cost of services to the plan sponsor over time. Medicare is a defined benefit health insurance program.
Defined Contribution	Individuals are entitled to benefits defined as a fixed dollar subsidy for the purchase of health insurance coverage. It is an alternative to the defined benefit structure. The defined contribution dollar amount may be determined in a variety of ways and need not be directly related to the price of health insurance.
Managed Competition	A system of structuring the market for health insurance under which, according to a set of rules, health plans compete for enrollees based on the price and quality of services provided.
Premium Support	A variation of the defined contribution approach under which the dollar subsidy is related to the price of health insurance coverage, and the dollar amount is computed to ensure that it is sufficient to purchase a specific set of benefits.

example, managed competition principles formed the basis of the 1994 Clinton administration health care reform proposal, under which individuals would have purchased health insurance through health alliances responsible for administering competition among health plans.

While the managed competition approach does not promote a totally deregulated health care system (hence the "managed"), it relies on markets and financial incentives to establish prices and benefits. This places it in contrast to approaches under which pricing and benefits are determined by the government, as is generally the case with the current Medicare program.

Under managed competition, private health plans would compete for enrollees within a set of rules established and overseen by the purchaser. The competition is intended to be based on both price and quality of health care delivery, as well as to a limited degree on benefit design, with the goal of obtaining "maximum value for money for the purchaser and consumer." The rules of participation by plans (management of the competition) stipulated by the purchaser are intended to ensure that plans do not compete by selecting risk: attracting the healthiest, lowest-cost enrollees while avoiding the sickest, highest-cost enrollees. Without attention to this concern, all plans would work to attract healthy enrollees and avoid unhealthy ones; plans with higher-risk enrollees would be at a competitive disadvantage and might fail financially. All plans would offer the same minimum set of benefits to permit comparisons across plans and to minimize risk selection on the basis of benefit design. The premium paid by plan sponsors (employers or perhaps Medicare) would be set to ensure that enrollees have financial incentives to choose low-cost health plans. For example, a sponsor might elect to pay an amount equal to the premium of the lowest-priced plan. Enrollees choosing that plan would pay nothing; those choosing another, more expensive plan would pay the excess amount.

One of the biggest challenges in a managed competition approach is correcting for the unequal distribution of healthy and unhealthy enrollees across plans by a "risk adjustment" mechanism. Even with standardized benefits and other oversight efforts to prevent plans from actively seeking healthier enrollees, some plans still may have healthier enrollees and therefore look more efficient than others even when they are not. Risk adjustments modify payments to plans to correct such inequities and ensure that plan prices reflect differences in the efficiency and quality of the plan's health care delivery system and not in the characteristics of enrollees. With risk adjustments in effect, plans with less risky enrollees are paid less than those with higher-risk enrollees.

As a technical matter, identifying and measuring what distinguishes high-risk patients from others has proved difficult. Demographic characteristics such as age and gender are relatively easy to obtain but explain very little of the variation in health care use. More detailed information on the health status of individual enrollees permits better adjustments; nonetheless, the development of appropriate risk adjustment techniques is considered to be in its early stages.[2]

DEFINED CONTRIBUTION AND PREMIUM SUPPORT APPROACHES TO REFORM

The "defined contribution" approach to Medicare reform builds on managed competition principles. In general, Medicare beneficiaries would be given a subsidy to purchase coverage among competing plans. Converting Medicare from a "defined benefit" health plan to a "defined contribution" structure would make a profound and fundamental change in the nature of the program.

Because the defined contribution concept has influenced the development—and criticism—of recent legislative proposals, it therefore bears review before turning to the specifics of these proposals.

The terms "defined benefit" and "defined contribution" come from the realm of employer pension benefits, within which defined contribution plans have become more popular over the past twenty-five years. In the more traditional defined benefit pension program, benefits are computed according to a formula, perhaps based on years of service and percentage of pay, and are generally paid out as an annuity to provide guaranteed income in retirement. In contrast, defined contribution plans are employee benefit programs that are often designed more as savings vehicles than retirement plans. Employers pay predetermined amounts, typically a percentage of compensation, into individual accounts. While both plans have advantages and disadvantages, the defined contribution approach is generally thought to provide less security of retirement income because employee contributions or investment growth may be inadequate.[3]

Under the basic version of a defined contribution approach for Medicare, the federal government would provide Medicare beneficiaries with a subsidy, or voucher, toward the purchase of private health insurance rather than guaranteeing payment for specific health care benefits.[4] The voucher would not necessarily be given directly to beneficiaries for the purpose of purchasing insurance. Instead, the government could send the subsidy payment to the beneficiary's private health insurance plan of choice, with the beneficiary responsible for paying any premium amount charged above the value of the subsidy. Critical details of such an approach include how much the government subsidy would be worth, at what rate the subsidy would grow over time, the extent to which benefits could vary among competing plans, and what other rules, if any, would cover the private health insurance plans available for purchase with the subsidy.[5]

An important issue to be addressed in considering the conversion of Medicare into a defined contribution plan is the treatment of the original fee-for-service Medicare program (defined under the Social Security Act as "original Medicare"). While more than 6 million beneficiaries are currently participating in Medicare through health maintenance organizations (HMOs) and other private plans, about 85 percent of the program's beneficiaries receive their services through original Medicare. (Beneficiaries in original Medicare are free to choose their health care provider, and the provider is generally paid a fee established by the Medicare program for each service provided. Beneficiaries who are enrolled in HMOs are generally restricted to providers who are employed by or under contract to the HMO. Rather than being paid separately for each specific service, HMOs sometimes pay providers a monthly, per enrollee fee.)

In theory, under the purest form of a defined contribution approach for Medicare, competition would attract the participation of private plans, making them available everywhere. Thus, the traditional government-run plan could be scrapped, with beneficiaries enrolled in the private plan of their choice. Alternatively, original Medicare could be continued only in those areas that have no private plans available (for example, rural areas), it could be maintained as a competing plan option in all areas, or it could be retained for current beneficiaries, ultimately to be phased out as an option.

From the perspective of the federal budget, a defined contribution approach to Medicare has obvious benefits. For the first time, Medicare spending would be easily controllable and predictable for budgeting purposes. An annual aggregate Medicare budget could be easily converted into a per beneficiary subsidy amount. Or the value of the per beneficiary Medicare subsidy could be determined in a number of other ways intended to link it to the cost of the health insurance it is meant to subsidize.

Proponents of the defined contribution approach believe that it would lower the cost of providing Medicare benefits by creating a competitive insurance market. Beneficiaries would choose among a number of plans, which would compete for enrollees on the basis of premiums, benefits, and the quality of the health services they finance. Because the government contribution would be fixed, beneficiaries would have a financial incentive to choose the lowest-cost plan that met their health care needs. In such a market, plans would become more efficient in order to attract enrollees, and this in turn would lower the overall cost of the Medicare program. In addition, this view holds that the systemic savings achieved through private plan competition would outweigh the new costs to Medicare associated with competition, such as duplicative marketing campaigns and other administrative expenses borne by individual plans.

Underlying the argument that competition will improve the overall efficiency of Medicare is a belief that private plans, particularly managed care plans, will be more cost-effective than the original fee-for-service Medicare program. Managed care's emphasis on preventive care, discounting achieved through selective contracting, and utilization controls (for example, shortening hospital stays) are seen as efficiency advantages over fee-for-service systems. Included in this line of thinking is the notion that, in a reformed Medicare program, beneficiaries should only be allowed to participate in what is viewed as the relatively inefficient fee-for-service program if they are willing to pay more to do so, or if changes are made to original Medicare to make it more efficient and competitive with private managed care plans. The major concern with the defined contribution approach is the danger that it could "solve" Medicare's long-term financing problem simply by shifting costs onto Medicare beneficiaries, who then might not be able to afford the health care they need. Of course, the specific impact of a defined contribution approach would depend greatly on the details, particularly the generosity of the government contribution. But because enrollees would no longer be guaranteed any particular health care benefits, there would always be a risk that the subsidy would be insufficient to purchase comprehensive health insurance, causing some beneficiaries to forgo needed care. Even subsidies adequate to cover premiums for the lowest-cost-available plan might force those beneficiaries who cannot afford to pay more into a plan with benefits or quality of care that is not adequate to meet their health care needs or that would disrupt their existing care arrangements. If, as proponents argue, many plan options were made available across the country and appropriate attention was paid to quality standards for plans as well as to price competition, these concerns could be mitigated.

Furthermore, even if the level of the government subsidy was always sufficient to enable all beneficiaries to afford adequate coverage, a defined contribution plan would significantly change the relationship between beneficiaries and the Medicare program. In order for any competitive system to work, all beneficiaries would have to keep themselves informed about the health plans available to them and would have to learn how to evaluate their choices. Such a process would be new and confusing for many beneficiaries, and an aggressive program of beneficiary education would be essential. Language barriers and variation in literacy skills would need to be taken into account. Furthermore, unique aspects of dealing with the Medicare population need to be considered. Some elderly and disabled individuals have physical or cognitive limitations that would make it difficult if not impossible for them to participate as active and savvy consumers in the way envisioned under the defined contribution approach. Indeed, nearly one-quarter of Medicare beneficiaries have cognitive impairments.[6]

These issues surface in the Medicare program already since alternative plans are available to many beneficiaries, but they would become critical under a defined contribution approach. The worst-case scenario currently for beneficiaries who stay in original Medicare because they are unaware of or confused by the availability of other choices is that they pass up possible savings on additional benefits. Under the defined contribution approach, beneficiaries who did not understand the implications of various plan options could pay much more than they do currently for basic Medicare benefits or could be locked into a network of providers inadequate to their needs.

Beyond the issues of financing, shifting the locus of decision-making about health care coverage and payment is another aspect of a defined contribution approach that appears to be attractive to some policymakers. Under a subsidy program, many difficult decisions about coverage of new technologies as well as about how to constrain payments to health care providers or limit benefits to keep within available resources could be left to private health plans rather than to the government. The government could modify the formula under which its Medicare contribution is determined, but many other changes would be made by individual plans. Plans may raise premiums, modify benefits, or reduce payments to health care providers. Plans will make these decisions taking into account calculations such as the likely behavior of competing plans, how changes would affect provider participation in the plan, the likely effect on beneficiary enrollment decisions, and other market conditions. Like private plans, those responsible for operating the fee-for-service Medicare program would have to consider these elements in order to ensure its financial survival.

Concern about micromanagement of the Medicare program by both Congress and the Health Care Financing Administration (HCFA) is often raised by supporters of reform and seems to underlie the desire to shift the locus of decisionmaking away from the government to private plans.[7] This concern has been highlighted in recent years as efforts to slow growth in Medicare spending have produced complex policy decisions involving the creation and modification of fee schedules and other payment systems. All of these decisions are made within the context of the legislative and regulatory process, with the interests of beneficiaries, providers, and taxpayers in the balance, and they often have been the subject of intense congressional debate. At the same time that some policymakers may welcome relief from these hard choices, however, the push for increased regulation of managed care plans in most states and in Washington suggests that the public is not entirely comfortable granting private organizations sweeping authority to make decisions affecting access to health care services. At a more fundamental level than the popular desire for some government oversight of private health plans, policymakers will always be held accountable for how well the Medicare program serves beneficiaries because public dollars are involved.

As discussions about Medicare reform have evolved in Congress and policy circles, proposals for a defined contribution approach appear to have been set aside in favor of "premium support." The basic scheme of competing plans and providing beneficiaries with financial incentives to choose lower-cost plans is the same under both constructs. In at least one view, however, that of Robert Reischauer, "defined contribution" describes a system under which the amount the government pays toward private health plan premiums is calculated by formula and unrelated to the cost of health care benefits. For example, the government contribution could be computed simply to meet federal budgetary goals. In contrast, under a premium support approach, the dollar amount of the government contribution is linked in some way to the cost of a core set of benefits. This could be accomplished by basing contributions on the prices bid by competing plans for a basic set of benefits, for example.[8] With this distinction, premium support can be seen as a variation of a defined contribution approach that responds to the strongest criticisms about how a pure defined contribution approach would affect the ability of Medicare beneficiaries to pay for the health care services they need.

Plan Competition in Practice: The Federal Employees Health Benefits Program and Medicare+Choice

The Federal Employees Health Benefits Plan (FEHBP), through which federal employees receive their health insurance coverage, and Medicare+Choice, the part of Medicare that permits beneficiaries to receive coverage through private plans, each have been cited as models for reforming Medicare using competition among private plans. Experience with these programs is useful in identifying issues that must be confronted when considering approaches to increase Medicare's reliance on plan competition.

THE FEDERAL EMPLOYEES HEALTH BENEFITS PROGRAM AS A MODEL FOR MEDICARE

FEHBP is often suggested as a model for a reformed Medicare program. (Indeed, FEHBP has been offered as the basis for health care reform proposals involving the non-Medicare population as well.) Beyond the obvious political appeal of advocating that other Americans should have the same health insurance as members of Congress and federal employees, FEHBP is cited, with some overstatement, as a working model of the premium support approach to providing health insurance.

FEHBP does feature some elements of a premium support approach. Federal employees and retirees are provided an annual choice of private health plans, including a national Blue Cross/Blue Shield plan, several other national plans offered by federal employee associations, and a varying number of local HMOs.[9] The Office of Personnel Management, which contracts with plans, provides participants with comparative information on plan benefits, premiums, and quality measures.

The financing of FEHBP is somewhat reflective of premium support principles. The government contribution toward employee coverage provides some incentive for employees to choose lower-cost plans, consistent with the defined contribution and premium support approaches.[10] But under FEHBP, benefits vary across plans, and the government contribution is not linked to any specific set of guaranteed benefits. As described earlier, the emerging premium support model would have the government payment ensure that at least one plan offering a particular set of benefits would always be available for the minimum enrollee contribution.

One area in which FEHBP has not been a model for the managed competition or premium support approaches is in avoiding biased selection of plans. The program has had no mechanism for adjusting premiums among plans to reflect the relative risk of enrollees. The result is a wide variation in plan premiums, even within geographic areas, largely owing to differences in the characteristics of enrollees. This means that the government is most likely compensating excessively those plans that have enrolled relatively healthy enrollees and therefore overpaying for health benefits overall. For example, one analysis of the Washington, D.C., area found that while the estimated benefit value of plans varied by 31 percent, premiums varied by 159 percent, with the geographic basis on which premiums are computed and overall plan efficiency explaining little of the variation.[11]

A history of relatively low premium growth has been suggested as an advantage of the FEHBP approach, but, like private sector health costs generally, the trend more recently has gone in reverse. Spending per FEHBP enrollee grew at an annual rate of 7.1 percent over the 1987–97 period, compared with 8.1 percent growth in per capita spending under Medicare. While annual FEHBP spending growth was below this average in the mid-1990s, the past two years have seen sharper increases—premiums increased by an average of 7.2 percent in 1998, 9.5 percent in 1999, and 9.3 percent in 2000.[12] In contrast, Medicare spending growth has been much slower than average in the past few years, with an unprecedented decrease in 1999.

The important question is to what extent the structure of FEHBP demonstrates cost-containment success that could be replicated in Medicare. Proponents argue that the Office of Personnel Management (OPM) can use its administrative flexibility and bargaining power to negotiate favorable terms with plans. Other students of the FEHBP believe, however, that the OPM has been less active as a premium negotiator than is often suggested.[13] In addition, like any employer, the federal government is constrained in managing its health benefits program by having to take into account labor market conditions and likely employee reaction when considering any decision that might reduce benefits or require employees to leave a popular plan. Unlike for private sector employers, there is a political element as well, as unions and employee associations have recourse to Congress if they are unhappy with OPM decisions. These constraints are cited by analysts as making it difficult for OPM to avoid, for example, recent double-digit increases in the Blue Cross/Blue Shield premium, the most popular plan.[14]

How the virtues of this process could be applied to the Medicare program is uncertain. If the FEHBP model were directly adopted by Medicare, private plans would have freedom to propose benefits and premiums. But how much of a "free market" would be created is arguable given that the government, possessing new flexibility in entering into agreements with plans, would have a great deal of negotiating strength in representing the single largest pool of potential plan enrollees. On the other hand, the negotiating balance could shift if the FEHBP model were applied in its entirety and Medicare no longer operated its own health insurance program. Under that circumstance, the government would be responsible for arranging affordable private coverage options for millions of Medicare beneficiaries around the country without a safety net.

MEDICARE+CHOICE AS A PLATFORM FOR MEDICARE REFORM

The changing nature of HMOs and their role in the American health care system have been reflected in Medicare policies over the years. Only a small number of HMOs existed when the Medicare program began in the 1960s. Since these organizations were not set up to bill on a fee-for-service basis as Medicare generally requires, special policies were created to pay HMOs for services provided to Medicare beneficiaries. As managed care began to expand in the 1980s, a mechanism was established under which managed care plans could contract to provide Medicare benefits for a monthly, per enrollee (capitation) payment.

More recently, influenced by the managed competition model, major changes were made to the Medicare managed care program in 1997, with the creation of Medicare+Choice under the Balanced Budget Act of 1997 (BBA). More plan choices were encouraged, as private plans other than HMOs, such as provider-sponsored organizations, preferred provider organizations, and private fee-for-service plans, were enabled to participate in Medicare. An annual open enrollment process was established, consistent with the managed competition model, under which beneficiaries would ultimately be locked in yearly to their plan choices.

The most significant changes made under the BBA, however, were those regarding how plans are paid, and issues surrounding payments to Medicare+Choice plans are relevant to reform proposals based on increasing plan competition. They include the overall level of payments to plans, the related issue of risk adjustment methodology, and geographic variation in plan payments leading to differences in benefits.

Overall level of plan payments. Under pre-BBA policies, aggregate Medicare payments to HMOs were known to be excessive. Medicare had generally paid HMOs capitation rates based on the cost experience of fee-for-service Medicare in their local area, less 5 percent, a discount intended to recognize managed care efficiencies. For years, analysts have concluded that, despite this discount, plans are overpaid because beneficiaries choosing HMOs are relatively healthy compared with those enrolled in original Medicare.[15] While payments were adjusted to reflect cost differences attributable to demographic characteristics, such as age, sex, and institutionalization status, these adjustments were insufficient to correct for the relatively healthy condition of the Medicare HMO population. In response, the BBA lessened increases in average plan payments for several years and required adoption of a new risk adjustment system, although subsequent legislation reversed these to some extent.

Risk adjustment. Because risk adjustment is critical to the success of any plan competition approach, the associated operational difficulties are important to note. The new risk adjustment system resulting from the BBA requirements will be based on actual use of services by individual enrollees, initially using inpatient hospital data.[16] Plans will be paid more for enrollees who have in the past been hospitalized with certain diagnoses than they will for those enrollees who have not had such a hospital stay. The new system is controversial, in part because it will result in a reduction in total payments to Medicare+Choice plans. More important, since it reflects exclusively inpatient hospital data, it is considered only a first-generation risk adjustment system, one that may inadvertently encourage greater use of those services that trigger higher payment. HCFA has indicated that it plans to move to a more comprehensive risk adjustment system by 2004, but many technical obstacles must be overcome before then. In particular, plans must develop information-gathering procedures that enable them to furnish the accurate health status data necessary for such a system to work.

Geographic variations in payments and benefits. The BBA also made changes in payments to reduce geographic disparities among Medicare payments to managed care plans—a particularly complex issue because it has implications for the scope of benefit packages available to Medicare beneficiaries through Medicare+Choice plans. As will be seen in Chapter 3, all Medicare reform proposals will confront difficult choices involving geographic variation.

Specifically, in some high-cost areas, Medicare payments to Medicare+Choice plans have permitted HMOs to offer Medicare enrollees additional benefits, such as prescription drug coverage, for no additional premium. In other areas, payments to plans have not permitted as much additional coverage, or no private plan options were available at all. The opportunity that some Medicare beneficiaries have had to receive federally subsidized supplemental benefits might not seem to be a problem; in fact, it is arguably a good incentive to encourage beneficiaries to enroll in managed care plans, if that is seen as desirable.

But free additional coverage has not been uniformly on offer. Its availability depends on how much Medicare pays plans in an area, including overpayments resulting from favorable risk selection, rather than on the efficiency of the local HMOs. By modifying payments to plans (for example, increasing payments in rural areas and blending payment rates in high-cost areas with national average rates), the BBA policies intended to encourage HMOs to offer policies in previously unserved areas while attaining savings in places where overpayment has been a concern.

Medicare+Choice experience and lessons for Medicare reform. While both the number and proportion of beneficiaries opting to receive Medicare benefits through a Medicare+Choice plan have grown since the program began, expansion in Medicare+Choice enrollment has been less than expected, and the curve flattened in 2000. In January 1998, the Congressional Budget Office projected that, with the enactment of Medicare+Choice, enrollment in managed care plans would grow by about 20 percent a year—reaching 7.8 million in 2000 (about 20 percent of enrollees) and more than doubling to 16.8 million, or 38 percent of enrollees, by 2008.[17] As of July 2000, however, 6.2 million Medicare beneficiaries were enrolled in private plans (about 16 percent of beneficiaries). While this is significantly higher than the figures prior to implementation of Medicare+Choice (5.2 million enrollees for December 1997), plan enrollment fell during 2000—having peaked at 6.4 million in December 1999.[18]

In the past few years, Medicare+Choice plans have reduced the extra benefits that are a major attraction to enrollees. More plans are charging a premium for such benefits, and prescription drug coverage is being significantly reduced by caps and copayments.[19] The average premium for the basic benefit package for continuing plans rose from $5 a month in 1999 to $16 a month in 2000.[20] Plan withdrawals from the program also have been a concern, disrupting coverage for thousands of beneficiaries.[21] Even more plans intend to reduce benefits or withdraw from program participation in 2001.[22]

These changes have occurred despite continual findings that Medicare+Choice plans are overpaid for basic benefits, adding to the cost of the Medicare program. Unusually small increases in payments to plans over the past few years have been applied, indirectly reflecting savings achieved in the original Medicare program as well as changes in Medicare+Choice compensation policies. Coupled with the rising costs of prescription drug coverage, the amounts awarded apparently have not been sufficient for many plans to maintain the level of benefits that draw enrollees or for making Medicare+Choice participation an attractive line of business for plans. Thus, the Medicare+Choice program may inadvertently have achieved greater beneficiary equity by taking away the additional coverage provided to beneficiaries in some areas rather than by making those benefits more available to others, as intended. The 106th Congress enacted legislation to increase Medicare+Choice payments to plans in an attempt to reverse these trends.

This recent experience with Medicare+Choice sets the stage for the larger debate over the long-term role of private plans in Medicare. In the view of some analysts, difficulties with Medicare+Choice reveal the advantages of a premium support approach under which plans could bid premiums reflecting local market conditions rather than being forced to accept or reject a government-determined payment level. To others, however, the Medicare+Choice experience raises questions about the feasibility of increasing the role of private plans in Medicare. If a major goal of reform is to make Medicare more affordable to taxpayers in the long run, private plans must be able to provide Medicare benefits at a significantly lower cost than the original program, especially given the costs and burdens associated with managing an expanded competitive market (for example, risk adjustment and beneficiary education).

Thus, issues emerging from experience with the Federal Employees Health Benefits Program and Medicare+Choice, such as the effectiveness of plan competition as a cost-containment tool, the importance of risk adjustment, and geographic variation in benefits, will figure prominently in the discussion about reliance on private plans in Medicare. Chapter 3 examines how the two leading proposals for Medicare reform suggest handling these and other issues.

3

PREMIUM SUPPORT AND PRESIDENT CLINTON'S PROPOSAL FOR MEDICARE REFORM

Two major proposals for comprehensive Medicare reform were discussed during the 106th Congress. The Medicare Preservation and Improvement Act (S. 1895), introduced in November 1999 by Senators John Breaux and William Frist (R-Tenn.)and reintroduced in February of 2001 in he 107th Congess (S. 357) is an outgrowth of the Breaux-Thomas proposal considered by the National Bipartisan Commission on the Future of Medicare. President Clinton offered an alternative proposal, initially put forward in July 1999. Both plans are complex, leave some questions unanswered, and are likely to evolve further as the debate over the future of Medicare moves forward. While they have many important similarities—including an emphasis on expanding the role for competing private health plans—the proposals have meaningful distinctions, particularly with respect to the treatment of original Medicare. Thus, they raise different issues about how a reformed Medicare program would work for beneficiaries.

PREMIUM SUPPORT

The reform proposal introduced by Senators Breaux and Frist reflects the premium support approach favored by the Medicare Commission. It would make major changes in the structure of the

Medicare program to increase reliance on private health plans. A new formula for computing beneficiary contributions toward the cost of Medicare would encourage beneficiaries to enroll in low-cost plans for their Medicare benefits. A newly created, independent federal agency would take responsibility for computing the government premium contribution, enrolling beneficiaries, and all other aspects of managing the premium support program. Original Medicare would continue to be managed by the Health Care Financing Administration (HCFA) and would be offered as an option to all beneficiaries, in competition with private plans.

BENEFITS

Under the Breaux-Frist bill, Medicare beneficiaries would annually choose a Medicare plan that would cover at least the benefits provided under what is now Parts A and B of Medicare. (Enrollment in Part B would no longer be optional; most beneficiaries enroll in both Parts A and B in any case.) Standard and high-option benefit packages would be available. Each participating Medicare plan would be required to offer at least a high-option benefit package. HCFA would have to offer a separate standard plan covering only basic Medicare benefits as well as at least one high-option plan in each local area. Private plans also could offer a standard plan, with some flexibility to vary the cost-sharing requirements.

High-option benefits would consist of standard benefits plus stop-loss and prescription drug coverage. The stop-loss coverage would cap beneficiary deductibles and copayments for standard benefits (excluding prescription drug coverage) at $2000 in 2003, indexed to the average increase in Medicare expenditures per beneficiary in future years. Private plans would be free to design a prescription drug benefit, which would be required to have an actuarial value of $800 in 2003, with that value also indexed in future years to increases in the "reasonable cost" of prescription drugs, a measure not further defined in the legislation. (A subsequent bill by Senators Breaux and Frist introduced in June 2000 as S. 2807, reintroduced in the 107th Congress in similar form as S. 358, and presented as a first step toward Medicare reform, proposes a more specific drug benefit, and indexing is tied to per beneficiary drug costs.) While the private plan drug benefit is not detailed in S. 1895, elements of the drug benefit to be offered by HCFA as the high-option plan for original Medicare are specified in the bill. HCFA would be required to contract with any private organization willing to provide this benefit, and those organizations would accept the financial risk of managing the benefit within the budget provided. Organizations could contract to offer the benefit on a national, regional, or local basis. Multiple high-option HCFA plans could therefore be available in some areas, depending on the number of contracting organizations.

The high-option plan would be available to beneficiaries for an additional premium, a portion of which would be subsidized based on income. Beneficiaries with incomes below 135 percent of the federal poverty level ($11,273 in 2000 for an individual; $15,187 for a couple) would receive a subsidy ("discount") worth 100 percent of the lowest-cost high-option plan offered in their area. Beneficiaries with earnings of more than 150 percent of the federal poverty level would receive a discount worth 25 percent of the actuarial value of the drug benefit ($200 in 2003). Those with incomes between 135 percent and 150 percent of the poverty level would receive a discount of up to 50 percent on a sliding scale. The prescription drug premium discounts would be treated as taxable income, reducing the value of the subsidy for some beneficiaries.

The availability of high-option Medicare plans is intended to replace individual Medigap coverage, which would only be available for purchase or renewal to Medicare beneficiaries choosing the standard plan offered by HCFA. Presumably this prohibition is intended to give private plans more control over the total cost sharing borne by their enrollees. Economists argue that allowing beneficiaries to have supplemental coverage that eliminates cost sharing exposes Medicare to having to pay for unnecessary physician visits. By retaining some cost-sharing requirements, it would be expected that beneficiaries would use fewer services, and growth in program expenses would be reduced. While changes in Medicare might affect employer decisions about designing retiree health benefits, some beneficiaries could still have employer-based retiree plans that covered all cost sharing.

GOVERNMENT CONTRIBUTION TOWARD THE PREMIUM

Instead of the current Part B premium, how much a beneficiary would pay out-of-pocket for Medicare coverage would depend on the plan in which that person enrolls. (Any discussion about how premium contributions are calculated quickly becomes complex and may seem overly technical. The contribution formula, however, is the heart of the premium support model, and a complete understanding of the premium support and other plan competition approaches to Medicare reform requires attention to this aspect of the proposals.)

Under the Breaux-Frist approach, each plan would submit a premium bid. The government contribution toward a plan's premium would be based on a benchmark equal to the national average premium bid by plans for a required set of core benefits, weighted by the number of beneficiaries enrolled in that plan in the previous year. Beneficiaries choosing low-cost plans (those with premiums up to 85 percent of the national weighted average premium) would have the entire premium paid on their behalf (see "Examples of Beneficiary Contribution under the Breaux-Frist Bill"). Those choosing plans with a premium between 85 percent and 100 percent of the national weighted average would pay a premium representing 80 percent of the amount above 85 percent of the national average. Those choosing relatively high-cost plans (those above the national average premium) would pay a premium equal to 12 percent of the national average premium plus 100 percent of the premium in excess of the national average. The 12 percent minimum beneficiary contribution specified in the legislation is apparently intended to match the expected value of the Part B premium contributions as a percentage of total benefits under current law, but the Medicare actuary has stated that, under subsequent forecasts, 9.8 percent would be sufficient for this purpose.[1]

Rural areas pose particular challenges under premium support. Currently, Medicare+Choice plans are generally not offered to beneficiaries in rural areas. Advocates of premium support expect rural areas to be more attractive to private plans than they are under Medicare+Choice because plans will be setting their own premiums rather than facing a government-determined price. Despite this change, some plans might not find it cost-effective to establish and maintain plans and provider networks in rural areas with relatively few enrollees or health care providers. Under the Breaux-Frist bill, in areas for which no private plans offer Medicare coverage, beneficiaries would be enrolled in original Medicare. In such cases, however, beneficiaries would not pay more than 12 percent of the national average weighted premium, regardless of the actual premium for the plan. If only one private plan is offered in an area in addition to original Medicare, however, the basic rules would apply, and

EXAMPLES OF BENEFICIARY CONTRIBUTIONS
UNDER THE BREAUX-FRIST BILL

If total premium bid by plan is:	Beneficiary contribution is:[a]
85 percent of the national weighted average premium or less	$0 (i.e., government contribution covers the full premium)
Between 85 and 100 percent of the national weighted average premium	80 percent of the amount of the premium above the 85 percent benchmark
Above the national weighted average premium	12 percent of the national weighted average premium plus the full amount by which the premium bid exceeds the national average premium
Examples if national average premium is $5,000 (85 percent of the national average premium = $4,250)	Beneficiary contribution is:[a]
Plan A premium bid is $3,000 (Plan A is less than 85 percent of the national average premium [$3,000 < $4,250])	Beneficiary pays $0 (government pays the full $3,000)
Plan B premium bid is $4,500 (Plan B is between 85 and 100 percent of the national average premium [$4,500 = 90 percent of $5,000])	Beneficiary pays $200 (80 percent of [$4,500 − $4,250] = 0.8 × $250 = $200)
Plan C premium bid is $7,500 (Plan C is above the national weighted average premium [$7,500 > $5,000])	Beneficiary pays $3,100 (12 percent of $5,000 plus $7,500 − $5,000 = $600 + $2,500)

[a] Exceptions: If original Medicare is the only plan offered in the area, the premium may not exceed 12 percent of the national average premium. Beneficiaries with incomes at or below 146 percent of poverty pay nothing for the lowest-priced high-option plan offered in their area.

beneficiaries would be required to pay any additional amounts depending on the premiums of the two plans. Rather than the current, fixed Part B premium, the cost to beneficiaries of enrolling in original Medicare would depend on how its premium bid compared to the benchmark. That is, original Medicare would be treated like any competing plan in this respect.

The extent of the government's contribution, and therefore any government savings generated under premium support, depends on both the level of plan premiums and the enrollment patterns of beneficiaries. Beneficiaries would be expected to choose a lower-cost plan as a way to reduce or eliminate their premium, assuming they anticipate receiving good quality care under the plan. To the extent this happens, the weighted average premium would decline, and the government contribution along with it, increasing the incentive for high-cost plans to offer more competitive premiums and further encouraging beneficiaries to switch to lower-cost plans.

GEOGRAPHIC AND RISK ADJUSTMENTS

Payments to plans by the government would be subject to both geographic and risk adjustments. As discussed in Chapter 2, improving risk adjustment is a key to the success of any health system that relies on plan competition, including premium support. The Breaux-Frist bill does not specify the details of risk adjustment, which would be a responsibility of a newly created Medicare Board.

With respect to geographic adjustments, the Breaux-Frist bill would permit adjustments only for variation in the "input" costs used to produce Medicare benefits in different geographic areas. That is, variation in costs arising from differences in patterns of use of health care services would not be recognized. As a result, beneficiaries in areas that historically have had higher health care utilization would pay more for their Medicare benefits, unless those patterns shifted. In addition, competition among plans offered locally versus those offered nationally (like the HCFA standard plan, original Medicare) would be complicated. For example, a local plan offered in a low-utilization area would have an advantage over a national plan offered in that area because the premium of the national plan would have to reflect the cost of services provided in higher-utilization areas. Conversely, everything else being equal, a national plan would have a competitive advantage over a local plan offered only in an area where health services are used with high frequency.

BENEFICIARY PREMIUMS

From the beneficiary perspective, one of the biggest changes in Medicare under the competitive premium system would be the higher costs for basic Medicare benefits that could result from the change in program financing. Currently, beneficiaries pay the monthly Part B premium, the cost of any private supplemental insurance coverage they purchase, and whatever cost sharing is not covered by supplemental coverage. Beneficiaries may have the option of subscribing to a Medicare+Choice plan, which could reduce their cost sharing or the burden of supplemental coverage and expand their benefits, but enrollment in Medicare+Choice does not affect the cost of their basic Medicare benefits, which remains the same Part B premium regardless of plan choice.

Under premium support, a beneficiary's choice of plan would affect the cost of basic Medicare as well as supplemental coverage. Beneficiaries choosing a plan that costs more than the federal contribution would pay more for their basic Medicare benefits than under current law. (Beneficiaries might make such a choice if it was the only plan in which their physician participated, for example.) On the other hand, beneficiaries choosing a low-cost plan might pay less than the current Part B premium or no premium at all.

While new plan choices might become available, the cost of original Medicare would increase under premium support. For several reasons, the HCFA plans would be relatively expensive. First, sicker beneficiaries already enrolled in original Medicare would be less likely to switch into a private plan, and the science of risk adjustment is not yet sufficiently advanced to recognize completely the additional costs associated with higher-risk beneficiaries. In addition, because original Medicare is a fee-for-service model rather than an HMO, fewer utilization restrictions apply. Currently, more than 80 percent of beneficiaries are enrolled in original Medicare, so the premiums of the HCFA plans are likely to weigh heavily in the computation of the average premium used to determine the government contribution for the foreseeable future. But because lower-cost plans also will be averaged in from the start, the premium for original Medicare will increase.

The availability of both high-option and standard plans and the lack of standardized benefits would complicate choices for many beneficiaries and could lead to risk selection. Less expensive standard plans would generally not offer prescription drug or stop-loss coverage and would be most attractive to beneficiaries who did not expect to use these benefits in the coming year or who have other supplemental coverage, such as a retiree health plan. Those who currently purchase supplemental coverage to limit their exposure to Medicare cost sharing or for prescription drug coverage would find the high-option plans closer to their current benefits. Thus, the difference in premium levels between standard and high-option plans might be widened because healthier beneficiaries chose standard coverage while sicker beneficiaries chose high-option plans. This would be especially complicated with respect to original Medicare since HCFA would have to offer both standard and high-option plans to individuals for whom individual Medigap coverage also is available as an option. (In S. 2807, beneficiaries would be required to make a onetime decision on whether to opt for prescription drug coverage, in order to minimize such risk selection.)

Low-income beneficiaries would have fewer options than others because they could obtain a full subsidy for their Medicare coverage only if they chose the lowest-cost high-option plan available in their area. Each year, states would be responsible for identifying low-income beneficiaries and for notifying the board of the beneficiary's choice of plan. States would continue to help pay for premiums and cost sharing for low-income beneficiaries, as they do through the Medicaid program under current law. And, as under current law, only individuals identified by their state would be eligible for subsidies. Any income-eligible beneficiaries not identified by the state would be left to seek affordable plans without subsidy.

PROGRAM ADMINISTRATION

As proposed, the Breaux-Frist premium support system would overhaul the administration of Medicare. The major change would be the creation of an entirely new independent federal agency to administer the program. This step would require a reorganization of the Health Care Financing Administration as well.

A seven-member Medicare Board would oversee the entire program, with responsibility for a wide range of functions. Board members would serve for up to two seven-year terms and would be appointed by the president with Senate confirmation. The board's responsibilities would be broad in scope and would include determining eligibility and enrolling individuals in Medicare, managing the annual plan choice and enrollment process, contracting with HCFA and private organizations seeking to offer Medicare plans, paying plans for Medicare enrollees, ensuring that participating plans met program requirements, informing beneficiaries about the plan enrollment process and providing comparative analyses of plan choices available to them, and monitoring the financial solvency of the overall Medicare program. The board also would have the responsibility of overseeing the financial solvency of original Medicare, which, unlike other participating Medicare plans, would not be subject to state insurance laws.

Initial standards for participating plans such as those involving quality, marketing, and beneficiary appeals would be based on those in place for Medicare+Choice plans, but the Medicare Board would have authority to modify or eliminate existing regulatory requirements as well as institute new ones. The board would establish and finance multiple, local nonprofit organizations run primarily by Medicare beneficiaries called Medicare Consumer Coalitions. These organizations would be created to develop information and educate beneficiaries about how the Medicare program works and what plan options are available in their area.

In order to carry out these responsibilities, the board would be granted sweeping authority and, unlike HCFA, would be exempt from executive branch oversight. It could hold formal hearings, issue regulations, and contract with other organizations inside and outside of government to manage the program. It could hire staff without having to follow civil service laws. The budget of the board and its proposed regulations would not be subject to review by the Office of Management and Budget. Initial start-up would be financed entirely from the Medicare trust funds, but once the premium support system was under way, the board would levy fees on participating Medicare plans to finance its operations.

HCFA would continue to operate original Medicare, with both standard-option and high-option health plans required as offerings. The HCFA plans would have to be maintained as separate, self-sustaining lines of business. While contingency reserves and initial working capital would be provided (with board approval), premiums collected for each plan would generally have to be sufficient to cover expenditures. Like private plans, the HCFA-sponsored plans would be subject to approval under requirements set forth by the Medicare Board.

HCFA would be reorganized into two divisions, one of which, called the Division of HCFA-Sponsored Plans, would run original Medicare. (The other division would run Medicaid and the State Children's Health Insurance Program and would carry out other existing HCFA functions.) The Division of HCFA-Sponsored Plans would be required to submit an annual business plan to Congress outlining policies for operating original Medicare and possibly requesting legislative amendments. For the first six years that premium support was in effect, no changes could be made to the original Medicare program without congressional approval of the business plan.

FINANCING THE GOVERNMENT CONTRIBUTION

Under the Breaux-Frist bill, the structure of the Medicare trust funds would be modified, and funding for the program would no longer be automatic. That is, under certain circumstances, the continuation of Medicare funding would require a change in law.

All financing sources, including payroll taxes, beneficiary premiums, and general revenue funding, would be merged into a single Medicare trust fund, with a new limit on available general revenue. As is the case currently with Part B of the program, general revenue transfers would be made automatically as needed to meet the program's financial obligations. But the bill caps general revenue funding at 40 percent of program expenditures. If this cap were reached, additional legislation would need to be enacted either to increase revenue from the payroll tax, to raise beneficiary premiums by changing the government contribution formula, or to lift the 40 percent cap. Failure of the government to enact one of these steps would create a complicated legal situation since the individual entitlement to Medicare benefits would continue but the funding would be insufficient. General revenue currently accounts for roughly 30 percent of program expenditures.[2] New subsidies for prescription drug coverage also would be financed from general revenue.

While it seems politically unlikely that the program would not be financed under this circumstance, funding for Medicare could theoretically experience a shortfall. Under a combined trust fund structure, the pending insolvency of the Hospital Insurance Trust Fund would no longer serve as a key indicator of Medicare financing trends. The proposed legislative cap may be intended to play a similar role by forcing Congress to review Medicare's funding sources if general revenue subsidies are relied on increasingly. Arguably, however, Medicare is such a large part of the budget that such a review is inevitable as part of the normal congressional oversight of the budget.

MEDICARE'S BROADER ROLES

The premium support approach raises questions about how the government would continue its social roles in financing graduate medical education and providing assistance to facilities that form part of our safety net (roles outlined later in this chapter). The Breaux-Frist bill specifies that graduate medical education and "disproportionate-share" hospital functions would be made responsibilities of the part of HCFA that is not associated with the management of original Medicare. However, the bill does not change the existing legal requirement for original Medicare to pay providers additional amounts for these purposes, which presumably would have to be taken into account in HCFA's premium bids. No mention is made of current policies providing special assistance to rural hospitals and community health centers, which also would continue as requirements for original Medicare but not for private plans.

PRESIDENT CLINTON'S PROPOSAL FOR MEDICARE REFORM

Former President Clinton's proposal would make a number of changes intended to strengthen and modernize the Medicare program.[3] These include enhancing competition among private plans, adding prescription drug coverage and making other benefit changes, making changes to the fee-for-service program, and dedicating part of the expected future annual general revenue surplus to Medicare. The proposal would not change the administrative structure of Medicare, nor would it make changes to the program's supplementary social roles.

BENEFITS

A defined prescription drug benefit would be offered as an option by both original Medicare and all Medicare+Choice plans along with all other Medicare benefits under President Clinton's proposal. Upon enrollment, beneficiaries would have a onetime option to obtain prescription drug coverage. (A special enrollment option would be tendered to current beneficiaries when the benefit is first offered.)

When fully phased in, the drug benefit would cover half the cost of the first $5000 in prescription drugs purchased by a beneficiary, without applying any deductible. A catastrophic benefit would pay all prescription drug bills once a beneficiary has incurred very high out-of-pocket drug costs ($4,000 a year in 2002, indexed to drug price inflation thereafter). Beneficiary premiums would cover half the cost of the basic (noncatastrophic) drug coverage, with additional subsidies provided to low-income beneficiaries. All premiums and cost sharing would be covered for participants with incomes below 135 percent of the federal poverty level, and a reduced, sliding-scale premium would be applied to beneficiaries with incomes between 135 and 150 percent of the poverty level. (States would share in the cost of subsidizing drug coverage for beneficiaries with incomes below the poverty line, as under current policy; however, the Clinton plan proposes state-managed but federally funded assistance for those with incomes between 100 and 150 percent of the poverty level.)

Despite the addition of a prescription drug benefit, Medicare beneficiaries would still face the need for supplemental coverage under the administration's plan. Beneficiaries enrolled in original Medicare would continue to be exposed to unlimited deductibles and cost-sharing payments. The administration proposes development of a new, "low-cost" Medigap alternative plan that would provide a stop-loss cap on out-of-pocket costs along with reduced cost sharing. Premiums for this plan would likely be lower than for the existing Medigap options, which provide more extensive coverage of Medicare cost sharing. Combined with the basic Medicare benefit, such a supplemental policy could provide Medicare beneficiaries with a package more closely resembling those offered by private fee-for-service plans. The Congressional Budget Office estimates that substantial program savings could be generated if beneficiaries switched to such an alternative supplemental plan, on the expectation that beneficiaries would use fewer (presumably unnecessary) services when faced with certain cost-sharing requirements.[4]

COMPETITION AMONG PLANS

President Clinton proposes a "defined benefit competition" plan, which would use the current structure of Medicare+Choice but shift the basis of competition among plans. Rather than the current government-determined payment rates, plans would submit a bid for provision of Medicare benefits, and up to 15 percent of the bid price could reflect reductions in Medicare cost sharing. As is currently the case, Medicare+Choice plans could offer additional benefits for an extra premium.

The new twist on competition among Medicare+Choice plans is that beneficiaries enrolling in a low-cost plan would receive a cash benefit equal to 75 percent of the difference between the government's payment to the plan and the plan's premium. This amount is described in the Clinton proposal as a reduction to the beneficiary's Part B premium, but the mechanics of how beneficiaries would receive this rebate were not detailed.

Medicare would pay plans the premium they bid, up to a cap. The cap would be the higher of the current Medicare+Choice payment rate or 96 percent of the per capita cost of fee-for-service Medicare in the area. Plan payments would be adjusted to reflect the relative health risk associated with the plan's enrollee pool using health status information, based on hospitalization records.

By this construct, the Clinton plan suggests modifying the way payments to Medicare+Choice plans are adjusted for geographic differences. Local cost differences among plans would be fully reflected. (In contrast, under the formula currently in place, payments to high-cost areas are reduced by blending them with national average amounts.) Without this change, beneficiary premiums for Medicare+Choice plans in high-cost areas might exceed the cost of original Medicare, which reflects national average prices and utilization rates. Policies in effect to increase payments to plans in rural areas would be retained.

BENEFICIARY FINANCING

The Clinton plan would maintain the status quo for beneficiary financing with three exceptions. First, beneficiaries could reduce or eliminate their part B premium by enrolling in a low-cost Medicare+Choice plan, whereas a beneficiary choosing a more expensive plan would pay any premium charged above the cap. No changes in premium financing are proposed for beneficiaries choosing to enroll in original Medicare, however. Second, President Clinton's proposal would modify cost-sharing requirements to original Medicare by indexing the Part B deductible to inflation, requiring a copayment for clinical laboratory services, and eliminating cost-sharing requirements for preventive benefits. Cost-sharing reductions would be available through Medicare+Choice plans. Finally, all beneficiaries would be offered prescription drug coverage as a Medicare benefit for an additional premium, which would likely permit some beneficiaries to drop or switch their existing Medigap coverage.

NEW APPROACHES TO MEDICARE COST CONTAINMENT

A number of provisions included in President Clinton's reform proposal are intended to achieve savings in original Medicare through cost-containment methods that are used by private sector health plans. They include creation of options under which beneficiaries enrolled in original Medicare could have their cost sharing reduced if they chose certain providers or enrolled in special programs that would restrict their access to health care services. These could involve instituting care coordination and disease management services or identifying specific providers associated with lower cost sharing for certain services (called "preferred providers" or "centers of excellence"). By enrolling in a care coordination program, beneficiaries would have their Medicare benefits limited to those approved by the assigned care coordinator but would pay less in cost sharing for approved services. Disease management programs would offer patient monitoring and education to beneficiaries with specific conditions.

The design of these new options is outlined in the proposed legislation, with critical details left to be specified in future regulation. Much more flexibility would be given to the Secretary of Health and Human Services to implement than is usually permitted by Congress with respect to the Medicare program. For example, any of these options could be limited to certain geographic areas, certain types of providers, subgroups of beneficiaries, or any combination of all three. In addition, the proposal would require that a system of competitive pricing be used for certain services such as lab tests, medical equipment, and supplies.

The Clinton plan also proposes a variety of changes to fee-for-service payment schedules. These proposals are consistent with ongoing Medicare cost-containment efforts (for example, reducing payments for certain lab tests), although some proposed provisions would restore payment reductions legislated in the past.

SIGNIFICANT ISSUES IN COMPARING
MEDICARE REFORM PROPOSALS

The two major Medicare reform proposals have much in common, yet important distinctions remain. Both plans envision an increased role for private plan options. Both would introduce a prescription drug benefit, although benefit details vary in important ways. Finally, both plans address the issue of introducing more flexibility in the management of original Medicare. In that regard, President Clinton's proposal outlines a number of specific program changes, while the Breaux-Frist bill anticipates that HCFA would propose such changes in its business plan for original Medicare.

The two proposals would have a significantly different effect on the way in which beneficiaries would participate in Medicare and pay for their coverage, however. In general, the changes proposed in the Breaux/Frist approach are much more extensive, and more risky for beneficiaries, than those put forth by President Clinton. Under the two proposals, administration and oversight of the program would differ substantially, with the Breaux-Frist approach making major changes to program management. Both plans intend to ensure the long-term financial health of the Medicare program, but neither claims to have solved this problem completely.

HOW WOULD THE MEDICARE PROGRAM
CHANGE FOR BENEFICIARIES?

Under the two competing proposals, Medicare beneficiaries would have different responsibilities, involving both how much they would pay for benefits and what actions they would be expected to take in order to participate in the program. Particular issues arise with respect to low-income and other vulnerable populations.

Beneficiary financing. The bottom-line question from the beneficiaries' perspective is whether Medicare reform means they will have to pay more for their health benefits and, if so, how much? The answer depends to some degree on the choices beneficiaries make under either reform approach. As mentioned earlier, the Clinton proposal would require some increases in beneficiary cost sharing but would offer beneficiaries opportunities as well to reduce the Part B premium and cost sharing burdens and to obtain subsidized prescription drug coverage.

The authority for new cost-containment approaches in the Clinton proposal raises consideration of an important trade-off between controlling the growth of Medicare expenses and restricting beneficiary access to health care services. For example, use of disease management services could lower program spending but would significantly change the nature of the Medicare program for beneficiaries who are already enrolled since they would have coverage only for approved services. The Clinton proposal may not pursue cost-containment approaches as aggressively as might be required to achieve substantial savings. In making the trade-off, the Clinton proposal leans in favor of fewer beneficiary restrictions and therefore less savings. First, the cost-containment approaches would be merely authorized, not implemented. In addition, if put into effect, they would always be voluntary. Beneficiaries could choose whether or not to participate and could be permitted to enroll for as little as one month at a time. Accordingly, the Congressional Budget Office attributes relatively small savings to these provisions.

Like the Clinton plan, the Breaux-Frist bill would allow some beneficiaries to lower the premiums they pay for basic Medicare, but, unlike in the president's proposal, beneficiaries would pay considerably more for original Medicare if lower-cost plans were available in their area. The Medicare actuary has estimated that premiums for original Medicare would increase substantially under the Breaux-Frist premium support approach. All such estimates rely on assumptions that may change, but this estimate found that if the proportion of beneficiaries enrolled in original Medicare remained stable, premiums would increase by 25 percent or more.[5] If premium support works as expected, a sufficient number of beneficiaries will switch into lower-cost plans, decreasing the average premium used to compute the government contribution and thereby increasing the cost of original Medicare by even more than this illustrative estimate.

The future status of the fee-for-service program is uncertain under premium support. Original Medicare would be expected to function like a private entity, submitting premium bids for the high-option and standard plans and financing services with the revenue provided through premium payments from the Medicare Board and plan enrollees. As structured, the bill would permit one or more of these plans to become insolvent, although, realistically, further political assessment would likely precede any shutdown.

Premiums from one of the two publicly operated plans could not be used to cross-subsidize the other. Unlike private plans, original Medicare (both standard and high-option plans) would have to be offered everywhere in the country at the same premium. Thus, managers of the government plans would have to develop premium bids that on average produced sufficient revenue to cover costs, but they would not be able to adjust the premium bids to local market conditions. In some markets, private plans might underbid the national premium, either because the premium was high by local standards or simply because it made sense as a business move to attract enrollees.

While the status of original Medicare is uncertain under Breaux-Frist, the willingness of plans to participate in the competitive arrangement proposed by President Clinton remains an open question. Several attempts at demonstration programs for Medicare managed care that would test methods of operating a competitive bidding system and the various technical adjustments needed have failed to get off the ground. One of the concerns of health plans is their participation in a competitive bidding arrangement that excludes original Medicare—precisely the arrangement President Clinton's plan proposes.[6] Plans argue that including original Medicare in the competition is required for a "level playing field." The Clinton plan does, however, include new beneficiary incentives to enroll in low-cost plans that might be sufficient to attract greater participation than has been the case in earlier versions.

Beneficiary responsibilities. Education and information are critical to the success of any reform plan that counts on Medicare beneficiaries to evaluate and choose among competing health plans. For many Medicare beneficiaries, the choices already available under Medicare+Choice, or even in the less complex Medigap market, can be confusing. Even prior to enactment of Medicare+Choice, health insurance counselors who advise the elderly and disabled found that many beneficiaries unfamiliar with managed care did not understand the difference between original Medicare and HMOs. In addition, counselors reported that, once enrolled in Medicare HMOs, beneficiaries did not always understand plan requirements regarding choice of physicians.[7]

Because the Breaux-Frist plan relies heavily on beneficiaries evaluating choices and changing plans when it is to their advantage, the need for beneficiary information and education is greater than under Medicare+Choice, even with the changes proposed by President Clinton. Under the Clinton approach to competition, a beneficiary who ignored other plan options and stayed in original Medicare might miss out on a lower-cost plan. The same individual under a premium support system could end up paying much more to stay in original Medicare. While the Medicare Board would develop information and fund counseling centers, it is unclear whether this would be sufficient to ensure that all beneficiaries were in a position to make the best choice of health plan. Of particular concern are those beneficiaries with cognitive impairments or health conditions that make it difficult for them to be active participants in selecting a health plan.

Availability of plan choices. Giving beneficiaries sufficient plan choices is the key to any successful competitive plan. It is especially important under premium support, which significantly restructures the Medicare program in order to promote greater competition. In particular, a successful premium support system would require that more plans be made available to beneficiaries in rural areas and other underserved communities than has been the case to date under Medicare+Choice. Proponents of the Breaux/Frist type of premium support proposal argue that more private plans would participate in Medicare if plan payments were based on premium bids and were no longer set by formula. But the program would not work well in all areas if this did not occur. While the bill protects beneficiaries from higher premiums in those areas where original Medicare is the only option (by limiting the premium to no more than 12 percent of the national average), under Breaux-Frist the presence of just one other competing plan would be considered sufficient competition to raise the cost of original Medicare for beneficiaries in that area by eliminating the 12 percent limit.

In addition to the number of plan choices, capacity to expand enrollment could constrain beneficiary choice. Depending on the extent of the provider network, some plans may not be able to accept all the beneficiaries that choose to sign up. In that case, beneficiaries who elected to enroll in a low-cost plan but were shut out could end up paying more than they expected for their Medicare benefits.

Effects on vulnerable beneficiaries. In any plan-choice environment, low-income beneficiaries will be less active participants if their income limits the plan choices available to them. Health care costs are already a significant share of income for this population, and policies that effectively increase this burden could make health care unaffordable for some.

Low-income beneficiaries who do not qualify for full, wrap-around Medicaid benefits would be made better off under President Clinton's proposal because they would receive subsidized prescription drug coverage (all beneficiaries would receive a subsidy of at least 50 percent) and because they also could have their Part B premium reduced—increasing their take-home monthly Social Security income—if they chose to enroll in a low-cost Medicare+Choice plan. The temptation for some beneficiaries to increase their monthly Social Security payments by enrolling in a low-cost plan reinforces the need for a strong program of beneficiary information about Medicare+Choice options.

Under the Breaux Frist proposal, low-income beneficiaries would face fewer plan choices. Each year, these individuals would have to enroll in the lowest-cost high-option plan offered in their area in order to receive a full subsidy. Depending on which plan is lowest cost, this restriction would most likely require some beneficiaries to change doctors. Because the enrollment process is annual, these individuals could be compelled to change plans, and perhaps switch doctors, in any year in which the plan identified as lowest cost changes, or could be faced with paying a higher amount, which might not be affordable. Being forced to switch providers would be especially burdensome for chronically ill beneficiaries or others in the midst of a treatment plan. Moreover, even near-poor beneficiaries who are not limited by the formal requirements would effectively have fewer choices because they might not be able to afford to enroll in a plan that would cover visits to their current physician.

Subsidizing low-income beneficiaries fully only when they enroll in the lowest-cost plan raises several concerns.[8] Capacity issues would have to be confronted: What if the lowest-cost plan could not accommodate all eligible low-income enrollees? What would happen to other (nonsubsidized) beneficiaries who wanted to enroll in this plan? Moreover, if all low-income beneficiaries are enrolled in the lowest-cost plan, it could encourage a kind of two-tier approach to Medicare benefits—a departure from the universal access provided under original Medicare.

FINANCIAL IMPACT ON MEDICARE

How successfully the Medicare reform proposals would work to preserve the long-term solvency of the program is difficult to estimate. In particular, assumptions about the extent to which competition reduces health care costs and whether managed care will continue to generate savings are critical.

Premium support. While there is general agreement among economists that competition among health plans would reduce the rate of growth in Medicare spending, the extent of the savings is a matter of controversy. The National Bipartisan Commission on the Future of Medicare staff estimated that a premium support proposal would, over the long run, rein in the pace of Medicare spending growth by 1 percent a year, accumulating to a 20 to 30 percent reduction in program spending by the year 2030.[9] This represents the optimistic end of the spectrum of estimates to date. During the commission's deliberations, the Medicare actuaries provided another estimate of the effects of a premium support approach. Under this estimate, total Medicare spending would be reduced by less than 12 percent by 2030, with premium support and fee-for-service modernization accounting for less than one-third of the total. The bulk of the savings was credited to other provisions in that proposal. These included extending reductions in payments to doctors and hospitals inaugurated under the Balanced Budget Act, requiring higher-income beneficiaries to pay more for their Medicare benefits, and increasing the age of eligibility to sixty-seven.[10] Perhaps a longer time horizon would have produced a different savings distribution, but the differences in the estimates highlight the degree of uncertainty with which policymakers are confronted in considering the premium support proposal.

The Congressional Budget Office (CBO) has not yet provided a cost estimate and analysis of the Breaux-Frist proposal. However, in its analysis of premium support provided to the Medicare Commission, the CBO indicated that introducing price competition among private plans would generate savings as more beneficiaries chose lower-cost plans.[11] Significant potential sources of savings identified by the CBO were, first, the participation of original Medicare as a competing plan with greater ability to manage its costs and, second, the geographic and risk adjustments as determined by the Medicare Board.

Over the long term, CBO stated that growth in Medicare spending under premium support should closely reflect private sector trends but hedged about what those trends might be. Analysts agree that, to some extent, managed care produces "onetime" savings, as individuals switch from more costly plans to HMOs. The ability of managed care to control growth in spending over a sustained period is less certain, however. [12] The recent increase in private sector premiums is not believed to forewarn a return to rampant health care spending growth, as employers and other purchasers are likely to continue to pressure plans and providers to restrain costs. The CBO noted in its analysis, however, that the success of Medicare premium support would depend on the quality of competition in the broader health care system, and a continued trend toward consolidation of health plans might reduce competitive pressures.

President Clinton's reform proposal. The Congressional Budget Office's July 2000 estimate of President Clinton's plan concluded that, if enacted, it would increase Medicare spending by $310 billion over ten years (2001–2010).[13] This estimate is the net result of adding the proposed new prescription drug benefit (+$297 billion), savings from the proposed competitive benefit approach (–$14 billion), and changes to fee-for-service Medicare (+$27 billion, including increased flexibility in cost-containment approaches saving $3 billion and new rules for beneficiary cost sharing saving $2 billion).

The CBO noted that the estimate for savings from expanding plan competition is "subject to great uncertainty." Put in context, these savings from competition are relatively small—the $14 billion is less than 0.5 percent of the total Medicare benefit payments CBO projects for the 2001–2010 period under current law. That amount would result from a total savings of $85 billion, offset by $71 billion in premium rebates to beneficiaries choosing lower-cost plans. The CBO expects that the administration's plan would increase plan competition in areas that have had few or no Medicare+Choice plans. However, it also stated that most beneficiaries would still be enrolled in original Medicare and that the savings from the Clinton approach to competition would be less than in the case of other strategies under which the original Medicare was in more direct competition with private plans. This last statement suggests that the CBO's estimated savings from a premium support competition approach might be greater than the $14 billion projected for the Clinton proposal.

MANAGING THE MEDICARE PROGRAM

By creating a new federal agency to manage Medicare, the Breaux-Frist bill would significantly change the administration and oversight of the program. Indeed, turning over the Medicare program—already 12 percent of the federal budget—to a new government authority with limited accountability is one of the more controversial and potentially risky aspects of the Breaux-Frist approach. As proposed, the Medicare Board would have a great deal of power to determine the future of Medicare. Many important details of the premium support system are not specified in the proposed legislation but instead are assigned to be worked out by the board. It would not be subject to executive branch oversight through the Office of Management and Budget, nor would it be required to justify an appropriations request before Congress since it would be funded by an assessment on participating health plans.

While a possible advantage of an independent agency is relative freedom from political influence, it also makes the selection of appropriate board members critical. Under the Breaux-Frist proposal, nominees would be subject to Senate confirmation, but the bill does not specify required or expected qualifications, or disqualifying characteristics, of board members, who could be removed only for neglect of duty or malfeasance. No financial disclosure requirements or restrictions on associations with participating Medicare plans during or after members' board service are included in the premium support legislation. Indeed, a board composed of representatives of vested interests (plans, providers) could reduce Medicare policymaking to a direct negotiation among stakeholders and, in the view of one expert, would "not take the politics out of Medicare. Rather, it would take the accountability out of politics."[14]

The introduction of the Medicare Board could increase the cost of administering the program. Currently, Medicare administration represents only about 2 percent of total program expenses. Under premium support, the administrative costs of operating original

Medicare would be maintained and financed through plan premiums. Presumably, funds to cover the continuation of those activities previously conducted by HCFA as part of its oversight of the Medicare+Choice program would be made available to the board. However, new costs would arise because establishing a separate agency would require overhead expenses, and the board would be carrying out a number of new activities that would require additional resources, such as notifying beneficiaries and the Internal Revenue Service about taxable benefits and funding Medicare Consumer Coalitions. Moreover, the seven board members would be paid more than the current HCFA administrator, and their exemption from having to follow civil service requirements in hiring could be expected to increase personnel costs further. Although the Medicare Board's administrative expenses would be financed through an assessment on plans, this levy would be passed along in the premiums charged by plans and therefore ultimately would be borne by beneficiaries and taxpayers.

A number of concerns appear to motivate the proposal to replace HCFA oversight of plans with the Medicare Board. At a minimum, the skills needed to operate a plan-competition program are seen as too different from those needed to operate the existing Medicare program.[15] Moreover, an equity issue is often raised—HCFA cannot be expected to oversee competition fairly among plans at the same time that it is running one of the competitors;[16] the suggestion is that it would bias the rules in favor of protecting original Medicare. HCFA also is perceived by many proponents of competition as engaging in excessive micromanagement and, in the words of one critic, being guilty of ". . . promiscuous promulgation of new regulations, rules operations, policy letters, procedural manuals, and other quasi-regulatory activities."[17] A Medicare Board, of course, could issue regulations as well and would do so with less accountability than HCFA, which must answer to both executive branch authorities and Congress.

The Breaux-Frist bill does not appear to achieve a "level playing field" between original Medicare and private plans, however. The disparity between original Medicare's national premium and the local premium bids permitted cuts against the notion of equal treatment of public and private plans. This setup makes the original Medicare plan a kind of default option for beneficiaries, which may very well be good policy but clearly puts original Medicare at a competitive disadvantage. Requirements that original Medicare provide additional payments to teaching hospitals and safety net providers also would unbalance the competition.

Furthermore, both original Medicare and private plans can be held accountable to beneficiaries through their market choices and the requirements of the board, but only original Medicare will always have an additional layer of accountability to the public through Congress. Business decisions by HCFA about what premium to charge, how much to pay providers, and how to design benefits would be subject to public scrutiny. For example, the Breaux-Frist bill places very specific requirements on how HCFA's high-option plan prescription drug benefit should be managed. For a number of years, Congress would have to vote to approve HCFA's entire business plan. While for at least one of those years expedited legislative procedures would be used, it is not clear what would happen if the business plan were not approved.

Finally, under premium support, there would not be any legal obligation for the federal government to continue funding original Medicare. If health care expenditures exceeded premium collections for either HCFA plan, it would be insolvent. The Breaux-Frist bill provides for a reserve fund to address these concerns, and future Congresses could choose to rescue the program from any financial difficulties. If, however, original Medicare ceased to exist, beneficiary choice would be limited across the country, and, for beneficiaries in rural areas, Congress would have to find a way to provide coverage if there were no private plans available.

Summary of Plan Comparison

While both the Breaux-Frist and Clinton proposals for Medicare reform include elements of plan competition, the approaches have different conceptual starting points, leading to a sharp contrast in the degree of change each would impose on the Medicare program, at least in the near term. President Clinton's proposal attempts to enhance the role of plan competition by building on the existing structure of Medicare+Choice and by providing beneficiaries with financial incentives to seek out lower-cost plans. The original Medicare program would generally be operated as it is currently, with additional authority to implement cost-containment strategies.

By comparison, the Breaux-Frist bill starts with a new construct for the administration and management of Medicare as a premium support plan and then fits the original Medicare program into the revamped competitive structure. This approach would establish plan competition as the centerpiece of Medicare by shifting the configuration of government and beneficiary financing, and it would provide no legal guarantee that original Medicare would continue to exist. General revenue financing would be capped under Breaux-Frist, while President Clinton's plan commits future general revenue funds to help finance Medicare.

The two proposals emphasize different time horizons. The Breaux-Frist plan would impose major changes on the Medicare program in the near term, despite the risk of unintended consequences, arguing that premium support needs to be put in place now to form Medicare's foundation for the future. It provides more limited subsidies for prescription drug coverage, arguing that the long-term financial soundness of the program should come before the expansion of benefits.

In contrast, President Clinton's plan takes steps toward longer-term program changes but puts priority on adding a universal prescription drug benefit to Medicare today, despite the added costs. Clinton argues that the federal budget can currently accommodate the costs, that the need for such coverage is great, and that competition among plans should be based on price and quality and not the availability of a prescription drug benefit.[18] Any additional program changes that may be needed to ensure the long-term financing of Medicare are left as future decisions, with the current structure of Medicare remaining in place.

OTHER POSSIBLE ELEMENTS OF MEDICARE REFORM

While various versions of private plan competition are the central feature of the current debate over Medicare reform, other significant changes have been contemplated. These include raising the age of eligibility for Medicare and finding sources of additional revenue. In keeping with the current congressional debate, the issues surrounding Medicare's additional social roles have not been a focus of this paper, but they will inevitably arise again in deliberations over the future of Medicare and therefore deserve a brief discussion here.

RAISING THE AGE OF MEDICARE ELIGIBILITY

Increasing the age of eligibility for Medicare has been in the mix of possible program reforms for some time. Most recently, the reform proposal voted on by the National Bipartisan Commission on the Future of Medicare contained such a provision. A phased-in increase in the normal retirement age for Social Security benefits from sixty-five to sixty-seven is already under way, and the commission and others have discussed raising the age of Medicare eligibility similarly as a way to alleviate the program's long-term financing problem. Improvements in the health conditions of older Americans generally and increased life expectancy might make such a change seem obvious, but postponing Medicare eligibility could easily add to the ranks of the uninsured. Health insurance is unavailable or unaffordable for many older workers and early retirees even now. To respond to the concern about loss of insurance coverage, the National Bipartisan Commission proposal would have allowed individuals ages sixty-five to sixty-seven to participate in Medicare, although no subsidies would be available to help cover the cost. President Clinton suggested allowing individuals ages sixty-two to sixty-five and displaced workers ages fifty-five and older to pay premiums to participate in Medicare, with a tax credit offered to subsidize in part their premiums. Both the buy-in opportunities and the age of eligibility will continue to be argued over as part of the debate on reforming Medicare.

FINDING ADDITIONAL LONG-TERM REVENUE

Even under optimistic assumptions, reforms based on premium competition, fee-for-service modernization, and increased contributions from beneficiaries themselves are not expected to solve the long-term financing needs of Medicare.[19] Unfortunately, options for finding additional revenue for Medicare—increasing the Medicare payroll tax or increasing general revenue subsidies by raising other taxes or incurring additional government debt— are unattractive to policymakers. Any tax increase is politically difficult; imposing a tax increase specifically for Medicare could be a particular challenge when millions of workers are uninsured. However, changes in the federal fiscal picture allow for a more optimistic scenario for the continued financing of Medicare. Indeed, President Clinton has proposed dedicating $115 billion of the projected budget surpluses for 2001–2010 to support Medicare.[20]

While setting aside some of the budget surplus for Medicare would be beneficial, dedicating near-term budgetary windfalls does not translate into long-term financing for Medicare.[21] The surplus funds the president proposes to set aside for the Medicare program through 2010 would not be needed in those years, during which Medicare's current financing structure is projected to be more than sufficient to pay for benefits. The money would be credited to Medicare's Hospital Insurance Trust Fund but used now to pay down the federal debt. Paying down the debt would lower the government's interest payment obligations and thus would be helpful to Medicare by reducing one of the competing obligations for future federal revenue. Medicare would be given a specific claim on these funds, but the question of how to meet the obligation to pay for Medicare benefits down the road would be left open since the trust fund transfer alone would neither generate additional future revenue nor reduce future expenditures.

Seeking to ensure the long-term financing of Medicare is clearly a worthy goal, and the desire to act sooner rather than later is appropriate, but there are limits to what can be guaranteed. While the demographic trends that will double the number of Medicare beneficiaries in the next thirty years may be unalterable, the uncertainty of estimates about revenue and expenditures thirty years from now should not be minimized. Forecasting the condition of the economy that many years in advance is tricky enough; once the complexity of predicting health care costs in light of technological advances and changes in the delivery of health care services is taken into account, estimates about the future become even more uncertain. At best, policymakers can work to set the program on a course that seems likely to succeed, given what we know today.

REEXAMINING MEDICARE'S BROADER ROLES

Besides financing health care services for its beneficiaries, Medicare plays other important roles in the health care system that arise when program reform is discussed. Medicare is the single largest purchaser of health services in the country, accounting for almost one-third of all spending for hospital care, 35 percent of home health expenditures, and 21 percent of spending on physician services in 1998.[22] Changes to Medicare can have profound reverberations throughout the health care delivery system, dubbed by one health care expert the "Medicare industrial complex."[23] In addition, the benefits of Medicare's administrative activities extend beyond the program itself. For example, the survey and certification of health care providers conducted to determine eligibility to participate in the original Medicare is a boon to private health plans, which can rely on Medicare participation as a guide in selecting their own providers.

Medicare also serves a critical role in financing the social costs of medical education and assistance to the uninsured and those living in medically underserved areas. Medicare's hospital payment policies make it the major source of support for graduate medical education in this country. About $3 billion in direct payments to cover resident salaries and $3.5 billion in add-on payments to cover the higher costs of caring for sicker patients in teaching hospitals are made each year. Moreover, Medicare further reinforces the safety net by subsidizing hospitals that provide health care services to the uninsured. These facilities taken together receive between $4 and $5 billion in extra "disproportionate share" payments from Medicare each year.[24] Finally, various Medicare payment policies provide additional funding to deal with the special needs of rural areas, where often a limited number of health care providers are available.

Reforms to Medicare could have serious implications for carrying out these vital functions. For example, can original Medicare afford to continue financing graduate medical education or rural health care needs if it must compete with private plans that do not bear these costs? Should these social costs be borne by Medicare alone, shared by Medicare and all other payers, or eliminated as a Medicare responsibility and taken up as a federal obligation elsewhere in the budget?

Indeed, these issues have already arisen in the context of Medicare+Choice. Medicare HMOs are free to choose providers and set the terms of their contracts and are under no obligation to help pay for medical education or the costs of the uninsured. Under Medicare+Choice, medical education payments are made directly to those providers who bear the costs and are not included in outlays for Medicare+Choice plans. Payments related to the disproportionate share adjustment reflect the fee-for-service program's acknowledgment of the provider's additional costs. These calculations are still built into payments to Medicare+Choice plans. However, these plans are not required to pass along the payments to eligible providers.

These important and difficult issues have been sidelined lately in favor of discussions about expanded Medicare benefits and the role of private plan competition. But as deliberations about the future of Medicare continue, expectations about the proper age of eligibility for benefits, the need for additional financing, and the impact of changes to Medicare on its social roles are all topics that will need to be revisited.

4

CONCLUSION

The Medicare reform plans offered by former President Clinton and Senators Breaux and Frist would both apply principles of market competition in pursuit of long-term financial sustainability of the program. The managed competition concept of encouraging multiple plan choices and offering individual beneficiaries financial incentives to choose lower-cost plans for their Medicare benefits is reflected in both proposals—but the underlying program structure would differ in ways that would be very important to determining how beneficiaries participate in Medicare.

For better or worse, the effects on the Medicare program and its beneficiaries of encouraging competition among health plans would be much greater under Breaux-Frist than under Clinton's reform proposal. That is, any savings from plan competition would be greater under the premium support approach, but so would be the risk of higher premiums and other demands on beneficiaries in evaluating complicated information. Moreover, these uncertainties are magnified in the Breaux-Frist approach because it would create a new, untested structure of administration and accountability for the Medicare program. In particular, the future of original Medicare, through which more than 85 percent of beneficiaries currently receive their benefits, would be far from secure if the Breaux-Frist premium support plan were adopted.

The fundamental question facing policymakers in evaluating the premium support approach is whether competition would generate sufficient savings to outweigh the risks posed by undertaking a major restructuring of the Medicare program. Future savings estimates from the Congressional Budget Office and others will be influential but not definitive, given the vagaries of predicting both the financial and the other wide-ranging effects of such a radically new approach to providing Medicare benefits.

Some advocates of premium support recently have suggested taking incremental measures. Senators Breaux and Frist have themselves introduced a separate bill intended to be a first step toward their vision of a reformed Medicare. Representative Bill Thomas, Senator Breaux's cochair on the National Bipartisan Commission on the Future of Medicare, authored incremental Medicare legislation (H.R. 4680) that passed the House in June 2000. The two bills differ, but they would both provide prescription drug coverage through private plans and would make changes to the governance of Medicare by creating a new authority to oversee plan competition. The Senate bill also would modify Medicare+Choice to allow plans to bid premium amounts and to share any savings with those beneficiaries choosing low-cost plans, provisions similar to President Clinton's proposal. While these smaller steps likely are a reflection of political constraints, their advocates may recognize as well that the reliance on developing more accurate measures of risk adjustment and resolution of other critical technical issues would make premium support difficult to implement in the near term.

Everyone is affected by Medicare, and not just because all Americans who live long enough will become beneficiaries. Younger Americans benefit from the success of the program, which provides access to health care for their parents and grandparents. As Medicare is the single largest purchaser of health care services, its policies have great impact on hospitals and health care providers that also serve the broader population. Indeed, a wide range of competing interests have a stake in the debate over the future of Medicare—current and future beneficiaries, taxpayers, private health plans, hospitals, physicians, and other providers in the field.

All of this suggests that reforming Medicare is likely to be an ongoing process rather than a single event. The history of the program suggests that whatever changes are made, large or small, are likely to be tweaked, unmade, or redesigned in the future. Until now, however, most changes to Medicare have focused primarily on how the program pays health care providers. The stakes are much higher when the debate is about changes whose consequences will be directly borne by beneficiaries.

NOTES

CHAPTER 1

1. Marilyn Moon, "What Medicare Has Meant to Older Americans," *Health Care Financing Review* 18, no. 2 (Winter 1996): 49.

2. Karen Davis, president, Commonwealth Fund, "Medicare Reform: Assuring Health and Economic Security for Beneficiaries," testimony before the Committee on the Budget, U.S. Senate, January 23, 1997, pp. 1, 8. Also, see *Medicare and the American Social Contract* (Washington, D.C.: National Academy of Social Insurance, February 1999), pp. 2–3, 20–23.

3. *How Americans Talk about Medicare Reform: The Public Voice* (Washington, D.C.: League of Women Voters, 1999), pp. 17–18.

4. *The Kaiser Family Foundation/Harvard University National Survey on Medicare Policy Options*, Henry J. Kaiser Family Foundation, Washington, D.C., October 1998, p. 8.

5. *2000 Annual Report of the Board of Trustees of the Federal Hospital Insurance Trust Fund*, Health Care Financing Administration, U.S. Department of Health and Human Services, report corrected April 20, 2000, p. 14.

6. Ibid., p. 17.

7. "National Health Expenditures: Aggregate, Per Capita, Percent Distribution, and Annual Percent Change by Source of Funds, Calendar Years 1960–98," Health Care Financing Administration, U.S. Department of Health and Human Services, May 7, 2000, available at http://www.hcfa.gov.

8. *The Budget and Economic Outlook: Fiscal Years 2001–2010*, Congressional Budget Office, January 2000, p. 87.

9. Medicare spending rose 3.2 percent for the first nine months of fiscal year 2000. *Monthly Budget Review*, Congressional Budget Office, July 11, 2000, p. 2.

10. Katharine Levit et al., "Health Spending in 1998: Signals of Change," *Health Affairs* 19, no. 1 (January/February 2000): 131.

11. *Budget and Economic Outlook,* p. 86.

12. *A Profile of Medicare: Chartbook*, Health Care Financing Administration, U.S. Department of Health and Human Services, May 1998, p. 49.

13. John A. Poisal and George S. Chulis, "Medicare Beneficiaries and Drug Coverage," *Health Affairs* 19, no. 2 (March/April 2000): 250.

14. Marilyn Moon, *Growth in Medicare Spending: What Will Beneficiaries Pay?* (Washington, D.C.: Urban Institute, January 1999).

15. Poisal and Chulis, "Medicare Beneficiaries and Drug Coverage," p. 250. Current enrollment figures from *Monthly Report: Medicare Managed Care Plans*, Health Care Financing Administration, U.S. Department of Health and Human Services, July 2000, available at www.hcfa.gov.

16. *Monthly Report: Medicare Managed Care Plans.*

17. "New Ratings: Supplemental Policies and Medicare HMOs," *Consumer Reports,* June 2000.

18. Patricia Neuman et al., "Understanding the Diverse Needs of the Medicare Population: Implications for Medicare Reform," *Journal of Aging and Social Policy* 10, no. 4 (1999): 36.

19. Judith Feder, "Medicare/Medicaid Dual Eligibles: Fiscal and Social Responsibility for Vulnerable Populations," Kaiser Commission on the Future of Medicaid, Henry J. Kaiser Family Foundation, Washington, D.C., May 1997, pp. 13–18. Also see "Managing Health Care for Dually Eligible Beneficiaries," in Physician Payment Review Commission, *Annual Report to Congress,* 1997, pp. 410–11.

CHAPTER 2

1. Alain C. Enthoven, "The History and Principles of Managed Competition," *Health Affairs,* Supplement (1993): 24–48.

2. "Risk Selection and Risk Adjustment in Medicare," in Physician Payment Review Commission *Annual Report to Congress,* 1996, pp. 255–79.

3. Kelly Olsen and Jack VanDerhei, "Defined Contribution Plan Dominance Grows across Sectors and Employer Sizes, While Mega Defined Benefit Plans Remain Strong,"in Dallas Salisbury, ed., *Retirement Prospects in a Defined Contribution World* (Washington, D.C.: Employee Benefits Research Institute, 1997), pp. 55–69.

4. Stuart M. Butler and Robert E. Moffit, "The FEHBP as a Model for a New Medicare Program," *Health Affairs* 14, no. 4 (Winter 1995): 47–61.

5. For a more complete discussion of technical issues in developing premium support, see Beth C. Fuchs and Lisa Potetz, "A Framework for Comparing Incremental and Premium Support Approaches," in Marilyn

Moon, ed., *Competition with Constraints* (Washington, D.C.: Urban Institute, February 2000), pp. 7–80.

6. "Medicare and the Cognitively Impaired," Henry J. Kaiser Family Foundation, Washington, D.C., June 30, 1999, p. 1.

7. Jeff Lemieux, senior economist, Progressive Policy Institute, "Building a New Medicare for the New Economy," testimony before the Committee on Finance, U.S. Senate, February 29, 2000.

8. Robert D. Reischauer, "Medicare: Beyond 2002," in Stuart H. Altman, Uwe Reinhardt, and David Shactman, eds., *Policy Options for Reforming the Medicare Program: Papers from the Princeton Conference on Medicare Reform* (Princeton, N.J.: Robert Wood Johnson Foundation, July 1997), pp. 102–3.

9. Mark Merlis, *Medicare Restructuring: The FEHBP Model*, Henry J. Kaiser Family Foundation, Menlo Park, Calif., February 1999, p. 9.

10. The government contribution is either 75 percent of the plan premium or 72 percent of the average of all plan premiums weighted by the number of enrollees, whichever is lower.

11. Merlis, *Medicare Restructuring*, pp. 39–42.

12. OPM news release, "Plan to Control Health Premiums for Federal Employees and Retirees Announced with Release of Premium Increase for 2000," U.S. Office of Personnel Management, September 20, 1999.

13. Mark Merlis, "Administration of a Medicare Premium Support Program," in Moon, *Competition with Constraints*, p. 88.

14. Merlis, *Medicare Restructuring*, p. v.

15. "Risk Selection and Risk Adjustment in Medicare."

16. *Report to Congress: Proposed Methods of Incorporating Health Status Risk Adjusters into Medicare+Choice Payments*, Health Care Financing Administration, U.S. Department of Health and Human Services, March 1, 1999.

17. *The Economic and Budget Outlook: Fiscal Years 1999–2008*, Congressional Budget Office, January 1998, p. 127.

18. *Monthly Report: Medicare Managed Care Plans.*

19. *Medicare+Choice: Changes for the Year 2000*, Health Care Financing Administration, U.S. Department of Health and Human Services, September 1999, pp. 3–10.

20. *Report to the Congress*, Medicare Payment Advisory Commission, March 2000, p. 120.

21. Mary A. Lashober et al., "Medicare HMO Withdrawals: What Happens to Beneficiaries?" *Health Affairs* 18, no. 6 (November/December 1999): 150–57.

22. "Medicare Refinements Should Continue to Improve Appropriateness of Provider Payments," statement of William J. Scanlon, director, Health Financing and Public Health Issues, U.S. General Accounting Office, before the Subcommittee on Health and the Environment, Committee on Commerce, U.S. House, July 19, 2000, p. 9.

CHAPTER 3

1. Unpublished memorandum from Office of the Actuary, Health Care Financing Administration, U.S. Department of Health and Human Services, February 23, 2000.

2. General revenue finances were about 75 percent of Medicare Part B, which represented 37 percent of total program outlays in fiscal year 1999. *Monthly Treasury Statement,* U.S. Treasury, October 27, 1999.

3. "The President's Plan to Modernize and Strengthen Medicare for the 21st Century: Detailed Description," Domestic Policy Council, National Economic Council, July 2, 1999; "Budget of the United States Government, Fiscal Year 2001: Mid-Session Review," Office of Management and Budget, June 26, 2000, pp. 1–3, 5.

4. *Budget Options* (Washington, D.C.: Congressional Budget Office, March 2000), pp. 228–29, 232.

5. Unpublished memorandum from Office of the Actuary, Health Care Financing Administration, U.S. Department of Health and Human Services, February 23, 2000.

6. Len Nichols, "Competitive Pricing by Medicare's Private Health Plans: Be Careful What You Wish for," in Moon, *Competition with Constraints,* pp. 105–18.

7. Frederick Schneider, *Lessons from the Front Line: Focus Group Study of Medicare Insurance Counselors* (Menlo Park, Calif.: Henry J. Kaiser Family Foundation, April 1998), pp. 16–20.

8. Merlis, *Medicare Restructuring,* pp. 69–71.

9. "Commission Staff Scoring of the Breaux-Thomas Medicare Reform Proposal," National Bipartisan Commission on the Future of Medicare, March 16, 1999, available at http://rs9.loc.gov/medicare.

10. "HCFA's Cost Estimate of the Breaux Proposal," National Bipartisan Commission on the Future of Medicare, February 23, 1999, available at http://rs9.loc.gov/medicare.

11. *A Preliminary Review of the Premium Support Model as a Foundation for Medicare Reform,* Congressional Budget Office, February 1999.

12. Sheila Smith et al., "The Next Ten Years of Health Care Spending: What Does the Future Hold?" *Health Affairs* 17, no. 5 (September/October 1998): 128–40.

13. "CBO's Analysis of the Health Insurance Initiatives in the Mid-Session Review," Congressional Budget Office, July 18, 2000. Also see "An Analysis of the President's Budgetary Proposals for Fiscal Year 2001," Congressional Budget Office, April 2000, pp. 43–59.

14. Judith Feder, professor and dean of policy studies, Georgetown University, testimony before the Committee on Finance, U.S. Senate, May 4, 2000.

15. Gail Wilensky, John M. Olin Senior Fellow, Project HOPE, testimony before the Committee on Finance, U.S. Senate, May 4, 2000.

16. Lemieux, "Building a New Medicare for the New Economy."

17. Sandra Mahkorn, "How Not to Reform Medicare: Lessons from the Medicare+Choice Experiment," Heritage Foundation Backgrounder no. 1319, Heritage Foundation, Washington, D.C., September 15, 1999, p. 2.

18. "President's Plan to Modernize and Strengthen Medicare for the 21st Century," p. 9.

19. "Final Breaux-Thomas Medicare Reform Proposal, *Building a Better Medicare for Today and Tomorrow*," National Bipartisan Commission on the Future of Medicare, March 16, 1999, available at http://rs9.loc.gov/medicare.

20. "Budget of the United States Government, Fiscal Year 2001: Mid-Session Review," p. 2.

21. *Analysis of the President's Budgetary Proposals for Fiscal Year 2001*, p. 68.

22. "Personal Health Care Expenditures, by Type of Expenditures and Source of Funds, Selected Calendar Years 1991–98," Health Care Financing Administration, U.S. Department of Health and Human Services, available at http://www.hcfa.gov.

23. Bruce C. Vladeck, "The Political Economy of Medicare," *Health Affairs* 18, no. 1 (January/February 1999): 24.

24. Congressional Budget Office, unpublished details of March 2000 baseline expenditures for Medicare.

Supplemental Insurance and Its Role in Medicare Reform

Thomas Rice

1

INTRODUCTION

This paper describes the current and future role of supplemental insurance coverage for Medicare beneficiaries. It examines how various Medicare reforms will affect the supplemental insurance market and, through that, senior citizens.

Because Medicare does not provide complete health insurance coverage, the vast majority of seniors have chosen to supplement it. The most common forms of supplementation are coverage provided by former and current employers, individually purchased "Medigap" coverage, Medicare managed care, and Medicaid benefits. Each of these, however, has its own shortcomings. Consequently, many observers have called for reform of Medicare and of the various forms of supplemental insurance.

Chapter 2 discusses the problems with the current Medicare benefits structure and examines the role of each major type of supplemental insurance, including both their strengths and shortcomings. Chapter 3 examines some important dynamics in the supplemental insurance market. It is necessary to consider how changes in Medicare or in any one form of supplementation will affect the program, other forms of supplementation, and—most important—Medicare beneficiaries. To give one example, to the extent that healthier beneficiaries join Medicare managed care plans, this results in a sicker group of people left in the fee-for-service component of the program, which in turn will raise premiums and result in more beneficiaries lacking coverage. Chapter 4 focuses on the potential effect on the supplemental insurance market of two alternative reforms that have received a great deal of attention: enhancing program benefits, for example, by providing coverage for outpatient prescription drugs and establishing a maximum on annual beneficiary out-of-pocket costs; and replacing the current Medicare benefits structure with one based on "premium support."

2

PROBLEMS WITH THE CURRENT
MEDICARE BENEFITS STRUCTURE

Although Medicare is often lauded for the excellent job it has done in providing necessary health care coverage for seniors, a strong argument can be made that the program nevertheless offers inadequate insurance. The primary purpose of insurance is to furnish a financial safeguard against large, unexpected losses. Although it might be desirable to have patients pay some upfront costs such as deductibles and coinsurance to keep down administrative costs and to reduce unnecessary utilization, good health insurance should provide nearly complete financial protection in the event of a major illness. Unfortunately, Medicare fails to do this. Consequently, most seniors feel compelled to obtain supplemental insurance coverage. Even though one often hears criticisms about the supplemental insurance market, it should be recognized that for most people possession of such coverage is a necessity.

Although Medicare does require some cost sharing (for example, in 2000, a $776 deductible for hospital stays and a $100 annual deductible for other medical services), the problem is that it does not suffice as protection in the event of a serious and costly illness. Under Part A (Hospital Insurance), patients face very high daily co-payments ($194–$388) in the unlikely event that they experience a hospitalization of more than 60 days and no coverage whatsoever if stays exceed 150 days. Under Part B (Supplemental Medical Insurance), there is no cap on out-of-pocket payments for the 20 percent coinsurance. Equally important, Medicare provides no coverage

for some other, potentially costly goods and services used by beneficiaries, particularly outpatient prescription drugs and long-term nursing home stays. This is why most program beneficiaries have
purchased supplemental coverage; it is also one of the reasons why
broader Medicare reform is attractive.

3

THE ROLE OF SUPPLEMENTAL INSURANCE AND ITS SHORTCOMINGS

In 1999, an estimated 91 percent of Medicare beneficiaries had supplemental coverage. Of this 91 percent, 27 percent had individually purchased Medigap coverage, 17 percent were enrolled in Medicare managed care programs, 36 percent (some of whom also owned a Medigap policy) had coverage from an employer or former employer, and 11 percent were covered by Medicaid.[1]

MEDIGAP COVERAGE

Medigap policies are designed to cover many of the gaps in Medicare coverage. In particular, they pay some or all of the deductibles and copayments associated with Part A or Part B services.

More so than almost any other type of insurance, Medigap has been subject to a great deal of federal regulation. In 1980 Congress passed the so-called Baucus Amendments, which required that Medigap policies contain certain minimum benefits, return a minimum percentage of premiums in the form of health service benefits, and provide various kinds of information to prospective purchasers.

Although the Baucus Amendments were deemed a success in reducing marketing abuses and ensuring that policies provided decent coverage,[2] a difficulty remained in that, with so many different configurations of benefits available, it was almost impossible for consumers to engage in effective comparison shopping. This problem was dealt with through the passage of the Omnibus Budget Reconciliation Act of 1990 (OBRA-90), which stipulated that all Medigap policies conform to one of ten particular sets of benefits.

There are still a number of concerns with the Medigap market. By providing first-dollar coverage, Medigap policies result in greater service usage and therefore higher health care costs; most of these extra costs are paid by Medicare, however, and not by the policy-holder through higher premiums.[3]

Another issue concerns the Medigap benefit structure. Some Medigap benefits, such as coverage of the $100 annual Part B deductible, seem unnecessary, and others do not appear to be worth the cost. For example, about 45 percent of Medigap owners have coverage for nonassigned physician services—physician charges above the Medicare approved fee—often at a substantial cost. This is unfortunate because program assignment rates are now well in excess of 90 percent, and physicians are prohibited from charging more than 15 percent above the Medicare fee schedule.[4]

The most critical limitation in Medigap is the lack of coverage for long-term care services. Such benefits can be purchased through a different vehicle—long-term care insurance. Those policies, however, tend to be even more expensive than Medigap policies unless they are purchased before a person is eligible for Medicare.

Because Medigap policies are expensive, they are not equitably distributed. The most popular policy, Plan F, with about 30 percent of the market, cost more than $1,000 annually in 1996 for a sixty-five-year-old and can cost much more for older beneficiaries. On average, Plan F premiums constituted about 8 percent of a seventy-five-year-old's total income that year.[5] The plans with prescription drug benefits are particularly expensive, not only because of this coverage but because beneficiaries with higher overall utilization tend to join. For example, the additional premiums associated with the Medigap plans that provide a maximum of $1,250 annually in prescription drug benefits average about $600 annually for a sixty-five-year-old, $1,000 for a seventy-five-year-old, and $1,300 for an eighty-five-year-old.[6]

Partly because of these costs, those who are better off are more likely to have Medigap coverage. It is estimated that in 1999, 12 percent of the poor and 11 percent of low-income seniors had no supplemental coverage of any kind, compared to 8 percent of middle-income and 6 percent of high-income seniors.[7]

There are other financial access issues as well. A growing number of companies use "attained-age" rating, whereby premiums rise as beneficiaries get older (though they start low at age sixty-five, so as to tempt them to join). Perhaps the key nonfinancial access issue is that disabled beneficiaries do not have the same open-enrollment privileges as seniors.

MEDICARE MANAGED CARE PLANS

Increasingly, beneficiaries are choosing to receive their supplemental benefits through Medicare managed care plans. These plans typically provide benefits in addition to those provided by Medicare; for example, more than 60 percent offer coverage for pharmaceuticals.[8] Although plans are allowed to charge a premium in addition to the Medicare Part B premium, most do not. In 1996, 63 percent of plans did not charge an extra premium. Among those that did, average charges were only about $150 a year, a small fraction of the costs of Medigap.[9] Thus, it has been possible to obtain many of the benefits of a Medigap policy with lower costs.

Growth in such plans has been rapid—almost fivefold—from 1.3 to 6.3 million beneficiaries between 1990 and 1998.[10] Although further growth is likely, enrollment has tapered off recently, mainly because many plans have pulled out from the market out of concern over reduced payments from the federal government. Between 1998 and 1999, the number of Medicare managed care plans fell from 346 to 310, and it was expected that only 269 would contract with Medicare in 2000.[11]

There is much debate in policy circles about the significance of the "managed care backlash."[12] Perhaps the main reason for such a backlash is concern that capitated health plans compromise on quality. Medicare managed care has not been immune from this criticism. One well-publicized study found that poor beneficiaries and those with chronic conditions had worse health care outcomes than those who remained in the traditional program.[13] However, a review of the literature shows little difference in quality and results between beneficiaries in managed care and those in fee-for-service.[14]

A second concern involves selection bias. Until now, healthier beneficiaries have tended to join Medicare managed care plans, leaving those who are, on average, in poorer health in the fee-for-service program.[15] The main reason is that seniors who are in poor health are more likely to have a relationship with a doctor that they want to preserve. The great advantage of the traditional Medicare program is that it offers beneficiaries almost complete freedom of provider choice, while Medicare managed care does not. A second reason for selection bias is that healthier beneficiaries are likely to be better informed than others and thus more likely to avail themselves of managed care options. Finally, although Medicare HMOs are required to accept all applicants, they have a strong incentive to aim their marketing toward those who are younger and healthier.

Selection bias is a problem for two reasons. First, it means that those who are sicker and who could most benefit from the coordinated care provided by some HMOs are less likely to enroll in them. Second, it drives up premiums for those who remain in fee-for-service, making Medigap coverage increasingly unaffordable.

EMPLOYER-SPONSORED POLICIES

Even more common than Medigap policies is coverage provided by employers and former employers. Because it is not individually purchased, such coverage escapes the extensive regulations to which Medigap coverage is subject, such as policy standardization.

Retirees with supplemental coverage from employers usually receive the same benefits as active employees. As a result, they tend to have lower cost-sharing requirements than those with just Medicare. Furthermore, because Medicare is usually the first payer and the employer provides "wraparound" coverage, premiums are lower than for Medigap.[16] To illustrate, in 1997 beneficiaries with employer coverage paid an average of $712 in premiums, compared to $1,249 for Medigap owners.[17] In addition, beneficiaries who enjoy employer-sponsored benefits have more comprehensive coverage. A full 86 percent have coverage for prescription drugs, while 29 percent of Medigap owners do.[18]

There are thus several advantages to employer-sponsored coverage over Medigap. Employers share in the cost and may be more effective than individuals in purchasing good coverage. Such protection is likely to be cheaper than individual coverage, irrespective of any subsidization by the employer, because insurers are less at risk when they insure a large pool of employees. But as with Medigap, there are problems as well, including the potential for high utilization of costly services.

One way in which the health insurance market has changed in recent years involves the growth of managed care. Most active employees who have job-based health insurance coverage are enrolled in some type of managed care: a health maintenance organization, preferred provider organization, or point-of-service plan. In part because they are familiar with managed care, many are receptive to enrolling in a Medicare managed care plan upon retirement. One recent study found that, among large employers, the percentage offering Medicare risk-based HMO plans rose from 7 percent in 1993 to 40 percent in 1998, although this has since leveled off.[19] Another study found that the percentage of firms offering retiree benefits in 1999 that provided a Medicare HMO option was 3 percent for firms with 200 to 999 employees, 11 percent for those with 1,000 to 4,999 employees, and 62 percent for firms with 5,000 or more employees.[20] These plans are often attractive to employers because of their cost-control potential and to retirees because of higher benefits and lower premiums.

One issue of concern is what happens when a senior becomes unhappy with his or her managed care plan. The 1997 Balanced Budget Amendment required that beneficiaries who enroll in a Medicare managed care plan at age sixty-five and who disenroll within one year must be allowed to enroll in any Medigap plan type (A–J) within sixty-three days of disenrollment. However, most beneficiaries are probably unaware of this law, and it does not cover a situation in which disenrollment occurs after one year has elapsed.

There is another, rather disturbing trend in employer-sponsored coverage for retirees: fewer firms are promising these benefits. One study reports that, among large employers, just 31 percent of Medicare-eligible retirees were offered health benefits from their former employer in 1997, compared to more than 50 percent in 1988.[21] When they are now offered, moreover, these policies typically feature more eligibility restrictions and higher costs for the retiree.

Employer-sponsored benefits are not secure largely because they are regulated through the Employee Retirement and Income Security Act (ERISA). Whereas ERISA provides various protections for the design and continuation of pension benefits, little is required of health benefits. Employers are free to cut or eliminate health benefits as they please.[22]

MEDICAID

There are four ways in which Medicare beneficiaries with low incomes can qualify for Medicaid coverage. First, under the traditional or "full-coverage" mechanism, Medicare beneficiaries who, because of low income or a disability, qualify for cash payments such as Supplementary Security Income or who are deemed to be medically needy because of their extensive medical costs can qualify for Medicaid benefits. The second route is the Qualified Medicare Beneficiary (QMB) program. To be eligible, a beneficiary's income must be at or below the poverty level ($8,292 for an individual and $11,100 for a couple). Third, the Specified Low-Income Medicare Beneficiary (SLMB) program is for those seniors with incomes just above the poverty level (not more than 20 percent higher). Finally, the Qualified Individuals (QI-1) program covers some individuals with incomes that are 20 to 35 percent higher than the poverty level.[23]

Of the 16.5 percent of Medicare beneficiaries who are dually covered by Medicaid, slightly more than half are enrolled under the traditional program, almost half are eligible through QMB, and 0.8 percent have SLMB.[24] Only a negligible percentage have QI-1. Like Medicaid for nonseniors, the costs of Medicaid are shared between the federal government and the state in which the beneficiary resides.

Those eligible for full Medicaid coverage do not have to pay the Medicare Part B premium, nor do they have to pay for any of Medicare's deductibles or copayments. In addition, they are eligible for other benefits provided by their state Medicaid program such as coverage for preventive services, prescription drugs, and long-term nursing home care. Beneficiaries with QMB do not receive these extra benefits but are exempt from paying the Part B premium and the Medicare deductibles and copayments. Those with SLMB and QI-1 do not receive extra coverage beyond Medicare; the benefit of these programs is that beneficiaries do not have to pay the Part B premium.

One of the problems with these Medicaid benefits is that eligibility is episodic: seniors go on and off depending on their income. One way to ensure continuous coverage is to purchase individual Medigap coverage, but this is very expensive and generally not recommended. Otherwise, when individuals lose their Medicaid eligibility they find themselves at considerable financial risk in light of Medicare's substantial premium and cost-sharing requirements and the age-adjusted premiums on individual Medigap policies.

Another major problem with Medicaid supplementation is that many individuals who are eligible for this coverage are unaware of this fact. It is estimated that between 1.9 and 2.4 million people are eligible for but not receiving QMB benefits, and 1.4 million are eligible for but not receiving SLMB. Altogether, this represents about 45 percent of eligibles. Just 5,000 of the half million people eligible for QI-1 have it,[25] although this is a very new program. Nevertheless, all of these figures are disturbing not only because these individuals are likely to receive less medical care but also because of the financial cost to them.[26] If someone is eligible for but not receiving QMB, SLMB, or QI-1, they receive $546 less annually in Social Security benefits because the Part B premium is withheld. Furthermore, those who should be receiving QMB are paying the substantial Medicare cost-sharing requirements or, alternatively, have a Medigap policy that they do not need.

Having Medicaid coverage makes a tremendous difference in how much a senior has to pay out-of-pocket for medical care. On average, in 1997 those with Medicaid paid a total of $337 per year out-of-pocket, compared to $1,735 for those with Medicare coverage only. Persons below the poverty level who have Medicaid pay an average of only 8 percent of their income toward medical expenses and insurance premiums, compared to 54 percent for poor beneficiaries who have Medigap coverage and 48 percent for those with HMO coverage.[27]

DYNAMICS OF THE SUPPLEMENTAL INSURANCE MARKET

Changes to the Medicare program will have a direct impact on each of the different types of Medicare supplementation. But even in the absence of such reforms, changes to one part of the supplemental insurance market can directly affect the other parts.

One such change concerns retiree benefits. Because these tend to be subsidized by employers, they are a boon to seniors who are fortunate enough to be eligible. Unfortunately, as noted above, we are now witnessing a significant retrenchment on the part of employers,[28] which is particularly disconcerting since it is happening during a period of relatively stable premiums. If, as appears now to be the case, employer health insurance costs begin rising significantly, it will be even more difficult for companies to continue to subsidize retiree benefits.

Where will these retirees go? A disproportionate number are likely to join Medicare managed care plans. Because this kind of coverage is cheaper, Medicare managed care plans are likely to be appealing. Others, however, will purchase Medigap coverage, and it is inevitable that still others will not purchase any additional coverage. As a result, the proportion of seniors with only traditional fee-for-service Medicare coverage likely will rise.

Another trend is the increase in Medigap premiums. In three states examined in a recent study, average Medigap premiums rose 26 percent in 1996. This was caused, in part, by the actions of the Prudential Insurance Company, which sold the popular Medigap policies for the American Association of Retired Persons. Prudential raised premiums by an average of 30 percent that year owing to a purported increase in claims volume.[29]

Rising premiums happen for a number of reasons, one of which is selection bias. One recent study found that Medicare beneficiaries in southern Florida who joined HMOs used 34 percent fewer hospital services in the previous year than those who remained in the Medicare fee-for-service system. It also examined those who disenrolled, finding that after leaving the Medicare HMO they used 80 percent more services than other fee-for-service enrollees.[30] Both of these patterns show evidence of favorable selection by individuals with few medical problems into Medicare managed care plans, and unfavorable selection for Medigap plans or other alternatives.

Eventually, this dynamic could create a premium "death spiral." As Medigap premiums rise, healthier beneficiaries drop out of the market since the coverage is not worth the cost. This, in turn, results in a sicker pool of Medigap policyholders, leading to higher premiums and more attrition from the supplemental market. Eventually, the group of people left in the market would be in such poor health that premiums would become exorbitant, and only the wealthiest people could afford this coverage.

Although such a scenario is possible, there is some doubt that it will come to pass.[31] Even though managed care plans have enjoyed favorable selection in the past, the future could be different, for two reasons. First, as managed care penetration rates increase, more of the working-age population is likely to be comfortable with HMOs and to be enrolled in managed care upon retirement. To the extent that this is a more random sample, more new Medicare beneficiaries of all states of health would be enrolling in managed care.

Second, Medicare managed care plans can potentially provide the greatest savings over Medigap for individuals with chronic health problems. In particular, through better coverage of prescription drugs, such individuals may be able to achieve substantial savings. In the future, this could induce sicker beneficiaries to enroll in managed care, thus reducing the extent of selection bias. If this occurred, then Medigap premiums would not rise so quickly, which should mean that the premium "death spiral" would not come to pass.

Perhaps the biggest unknown in considering the dynamics of supplemental coverage concerns the future of Medicaid coverage and other subsidies to poor senior citizens. This uncertainty is in part attributable to the difficulty of predicting the course of public policy with respect to these seniors. But it also is a result of the surprising difficulty of getting people to enroll in and utilize the benefits of coverage that is already available.

As mentioned, the key problem is that nearly half of those eligible for benefits do not receive them, mainly because they are unaware of their eligibility and how to enroll. Another problem is the challenge of getting dual-eligible seniors to enroll in Medicaid managed care plans. Although most states are emphasizing managed care as a way to control their Medicaid costs, currently there is no incentive for a Medicaid-eligible senior to join a managed care plan. This will make it increasingly difficult for states to control their Medicaid costs, which could result in other, more onerous cost-control mechanisms being employed such as paying providers even less or reducing coverage for optional services.

One distinct pattern embodied in all of these dynamics is that those who are most vulnerable in the future will be low-income individuals who have substantial needs for medical care services, particularly the near poor. Individual coverage is increasingly expensive and absorbs a large proportion of income; employer coverage is less available than previously (and has never been available to the vast majority of poorer seniors); and many cannot or do not enroll in Medicaid. Medicare managed care plans, many of which are available at no extra cost above the Part B premium, are an option for low-income seniors. There are, however, serious doubts about how well poor people with chronic illness can navigate their way through the system, given that the health plans and providers have strong incentives to control utilization.

4

ANTICIPATED IMPACT OF SELECTED MEDICARE REFORMS ON THE SUPPLEMENTAL INSURANCE MARKET

This section examines the implications of two alternative Medicare reforms on the supplemental insurance market: expanding Medicare's benefits and adopting a premium support program.

ENHANCED MEDICARE BENEFITS

Medicare's current benefit structure does not provide adequate financial protection to beneficiaries when they become ill and incur costly medical bills. For hospital services, Part A requires high daily copayments for long hospital stays; for Part B services, there is no limit to how much a patient can incur in terms of coinsurance for physician services. Nor is there any coverage for prescription drugs. As a result, beneficiaries are forced to purchase supplemental insurance in order to be safely protected.

One alternative that will be considered here is to enhance Medicare benefits so that such coverage is no longer necessary. Two enhancements are proposed: covering prescription drugs and establishing an annual maximum (for example, $2,000) on how much beneficiaries can pay out-of-pocket toward Medicare deductibles and coinsurance.

To enhance policy reference, this paper will model the drug benefit on former President Clinton's proposal, with one exception.

The president proposed a benefit that, when phased in, would cover 50 percent of prescription costs up to $5,000 a year (that is, the maximum Medicare payment would be $2,500). Premiums for this voluntary benefit would be $44 per month but would not be charged to beneficiaries with incomes below 135 percent of the poverty level. The one way in which the discussion below deviates from this proposal is that it substitutes a mandatory for a voluntary benefit since that is more consistent with the current Medicare program[1] and removes all issues surrounding adverse selection.

These changes would raise Medicare program spending; a financing plan is necessary but beyond the scope of this paper. Its importance should not be underestimated, however. Both of these program enhancements were part of the ill-fated Medicare Catastrophic Coverage Act, which was passed in the late 1980s but repealed just a year later.

In trying to predict the impact of changes in Medicare's benefits package, it should be kept in mind that supplemental insurance "wraps around" the Medicare benefits package. Thus, if Congress changes the former, providers of supplemental insurance tend to change the latter. In the case of prescription drugs, one would expect some Medigap carriers to cover all or part of the 50 percent drug coinsurance—assuming that regulations were altered so that such coverage was made part of some of the standardized Medigap policy types.

It would be reasonable to expect that Medigap insurers and state Medicaid programs would spend less on covering Part A and B services since beneficiary liabilities would be capped. They would, however, have to spend more by covering the cost-sharing requirements on prescription drugs.[2] How these two competing effects would balance out is hard to predict. If total costs to be paid by Medigap insurers went down, one would anticipate that this would be reflected over time in lower Medigap premiums.[3] State Medicaid programs would receive a windfall (assuming that their costs did indeed decline). The opposite would occur, of course, if their total costs rose.

One likely impact would be a decline in the demand for Medigap policies. Because Medicare would be providing better financial protection for serious illnesses, beneficiaries who could afford the out-of-pocket maximum would not be at risk of impoverishing themselves if they chose to self-insure (that is, having only Medicare as insurance). Thus, more people would feel secure enough to forgo supplemental coverage. Furthermore, by covering some of the costs associated with prescription drugs, the revised proposal would give beneficiaries somewhat more of a feeling of financial security. The prospective decline in Medigap sales, however, should not be overstated. As evidenced by the fact that 95 percent of Medigap owners have coverage for the Part A deductible,[4] one can surmise that most beneficiaries would not want to risk having to pay out-of-pocket costs up to the annual ceiling. And many are likely to seek coverage for part of the 50 percent coinsurance amount.

It is likely that these enhanced benefits also would reduce the demand for Medicare managed care plans. Two of the main attractions of these plans are that they offer prescription drug benefits and that they limit how much beneficiaries can spend out-of-pocket. If standard Medicare offers these benefits, it is likely that fewer beneficiaries would join HMOs. This would be especially true if plans continued to raise their premium levels above the monthly Part B amount.

It is more difficult to predict how employer-provided coverage would be affected. Although employer-based supplementation operates in various ways, the most common is the "carve out," where those eligible for Medicare face the employer's cost-sharing requirements rather than Medicare's.[5] Thus, the firm pays the difference between what it covers for its employees and what Medicare covers.

The two changes in the benefits package discussed here both are typically included in employer-sponsored health insurance coverage. Therefore, it is likely that employer costs for retiree coverage would decline, perhaps substantially. How, then, would employers respond? Almost certainly, those that are already providing retiree coverage would view this as a windfall; they would simply spend less on retiree benefits. More intriguing is what would happen to firms that do not offer this coverage or that had planned to drop it. The latter might consider retaining their coverage because their costs will have declined; this would be a very encouraging development in contrast to the steep downward trend in retiree benefits of late. There is a chance that some firms currently not offering retiree coverage would consider doing so if costs were lowered in this manner. That possibility seems remote, however, as firms face more powerful constituencies than their retired employees.

The impact of these options on the most vulnerable seniors—those with low incomes and those who have substantial medical needs—is likely to be fairly complicated. On the one hand, if Medicaid costs decline, as predicted above, then states could have more money available for such things as liberalizing eligibility, covering more optional services, or paying providers more. Similarly, declining Medigap premiums would make policies more affordable, although they would still be far above what most could afford. Perhaps the main effect would be on those without supplemental coverage. By capping out-of-pocket expenditures, the proposal would see to it that fewer people would find themselves bankrupt as a result of incurring large medical care costs, thereby making self-insurance a more affordable strategy.

PREMIUM SUPPORT PROGRAM

Adopting a premium support program would not only revamp Medicare as we know it; it also has the potential to alter the market for supplemental insurance substantially. Although a number of alternative plans have been suggested that differ in several ways, the basic idea can be described as follows.

Medicare would solicit premium bids from health plans, which would be financially at risk in the provision of program benefits. These bids would be required to cover all of the benefits that are part of the current Medicare benefits package but could include others as well. Medicare beneficiaries would be given the opportunity to choose one of these plans. In contrast to the current system, in which Medicare finances its benefits once the recipient pays the Part B premiums, under these proposals beneficiaries would receive "premium support" to purchase any of the plan choices available.[6]

Although the formula would have to be determined, take one hypothetical example: premium support at the level of 85 percent of the cost of the median-priced plan offered.[7] Suppose that the median plan costs $6,000 annually. Under this example the premium support provided by Medicare would be valued at $5,100. A person choosing a plan that cost $5,500 would be charged an annual premium of only $400, whereas one choosing a plan costing $7,000 would pay $1,900 to the health plan.

The main proposal for premium support is the Breaux-Frist bill, first introduced in the 106th Congress (S. 1895) and reintroduced in a similar form in the 107th Congress (S. 357). Under this proposal, HCFA would compete with private health plans to attract beneficiaries. Each would be required to offer a basic Medicare package containing the current Part A and B services as well as a "high option" that includes coverage for prescription drugs and also has a $2,000 annual out-of-pocket cap on current Part A and B expenses.

Under the Breaux-Frist proposal, health plans would submit bids for providing the standard and high-option benefit packages to a Medicare Board. Beneficiaries would receive a fixed "premium support" amount from Medicare and use that to pay for the plan they choose, whether it be offered by HCFA or by an approved private plan. Although the exact formula is somewhat complicated, in general, those choosing plans with lower premiums would pay less, and those who enroll in more expensive plans would have to pay more in premiums. Beneficiaries with incomes less than 135 percent of the poverty level would be required to pay no premiums for the lowest-cost high-option plan available in their area.

Enactment of a premium support bill most likely would result in more enrollment in Medicare managed care plans and a drop—perhaps a dramatic one—in the type of fee-for-service benefits provided by Medigap insurers. Its effects on employer-sponsored supplemental coverage and on Medicaid are harder to predict.

Under a premium support program all health plans wishing to enroll Medicare patients—including Medigap insurers—would attempt to compete for enrollees by offering an attractive benefits package at a competitive premium. Plans that could provide more benefits for lower costs would be favored so long as they were able to convince prospective enrollees that the quality of care they provide is acceptable. Until now, managed care plans such as Medicare HMOs have been able to provide an extensive benefit package at a much lower premium than have Medigap policies, so one would expect that many beneficiaries who are currently in the Medigap market would start to consider their managed care options—particularly once they had to pay the difference in premiums out-of-pocket.

Another reason to expect greater enrollment in managed care and less in the traditional fee-for-service program is that premium support proposals would end the implicit subsidy that is currently received by noncapitated supplemental insurance plans. Traditional supplemental insurance plans (that is, Medigap and employer-sponsored policies) are cheaper than they would be otherwise because Medicare pays most of the costs of the extra services that result from the ownership of these policies (which cover most patient cost-sharing requirements). Under a premium support plan, health plans that provide fee-for-service supplemental coverage would have to internalize these costs—something that capitated Medicare managed care plans have always had to do. Thus, if traditional Medigap insurers' provision of supplemental benefits resulted in clients using more services, then these costs would have to be reflected in the bids submitted by such health plans, making them less affordable and reducing demand.

It is not just Medigap insurers but employer health plans that receive this subsidy. Under the most common sort of arrangement, the "carve-out," members of these plans pay the employer's cost-sharing requirements, which tend to be lower than Medicare's. When this generates additional service usage, Medicare pays the majority of these costs.

Although different proposals vary, one aspect of some premium support proposals is that employers would provide retiree benefits to former workers by submitting bids to HCFA to cover the expense of caring for the medical needs of these individuals. By implicitly ending the subsidy employers now are receiving, these proposals create a strong possibility that costs for such coverage would go up.[8] Higher costs might indeed persuade some employers to forgo providing retiree coverage, aggravating the trend toward retrenchment by firms in recent years.

There are some other concerns about the employer market as well. First, some employers who have no experience in submitting capitated bids for retiree coverage could be so daunted by the task that they would simply forgo providing retiree coverage. If this turned out to be a serious concern, policymakers would need to consider whether employer-sponsored supplemental coverage should be excluded from the proposal. There is certainly precedent for this; none of the Medigap reforms in the 1980s and 1990s applied to employer-sponsored supplemental policies because they are subject to the federal ERISA rather than state regulation. Nevertheless, excluding such a large part of the supplemental market from the system would significantly dilute any efficiency gains that are achieved thereby.

Another concern is that the only affordable options for many retirees may be managed care plans. This raises some of the quality concerns previously noted. Still another issue regards selection bias. If Medicare is unable to implement an effective premium risk adjustment system, plans that manage to sign up healthier patients will be able to charge less. Such a case could result in a segmentation of

Medicare beneficiaries into distinct groups based on health status and perhaps income.[9]

Finally, consider the question of how the Breaux-Frist proposal would affect vulnerable seniors: those with low incomes and high medical expenses. The answer depends in large part on whether Medicaid is incorporated into the structured system of health plan choice. Under current law, there is no incentive for Medicaid-eligible seniors to join a managed care plan—they can receive care from any provider willing to treat them at zero premiums and with little or no cost sharing. One way to take advantage of any efficiencies that come about from managed care would be to include these low-income seniors in the Breaux-Frist proposal. This could be done by giving Medicaid-eligible seniors premium support from which they could choose a health plan. Those spending less than the premium support level would get a cash rebate, whereas people spending more would have to pay part of the premiums out of pocket. Presumably, many Medicaid recipients would opt for managed care.

This system would bring more low-income seniors into managed care. But one drawback of such a system is that, over time, the dollar amount of premium support might not keep up with health care inflation. (In this regard, the Breaux-Frist proposal is advantageous to the poor because it provides full coverage for at least one high-option plan for those below 135 percent of the poverty level.) If that were the case, then those on Medicaid might find themselves segmented into some of the plans that provide fewer benefits, or perhaps even lower-quality care. To be fair, however, there is no guarantee that the current Medicare system will do any better at keeping up with inflation either.

5

CONCLUSION

Because of the nature of the gaps in Medicare coverage, beneficiaries need to obtain supplemental coverage to have adequate financial protection in the event of a costly illness. Most beneficiaries have received this through coverage subsidized by a former employer or through the purchase of individual Medigap policies. More recently, many beneficiaries have turned to Medicare managed care plans because they tend to provide more benefits at lower costs than Medigap.

The market for supplemental insurance has been shaken by a variety of problems: rising Medigap premiums, a trend toward less coverage by employers, and the failure of millions of eligible low-income seniors to take advantage of subsidized benefits.

The first of the proposal types considered in this paper—enhancing Medicare benefits by capping out-of-pocket expenses and covering outpatient prescription drugs for all beneficiaries—would be a more desirable change for a variety of reasons. It would transform Medicare into a true insurance program, one that provides genuine financial protection in the event of illness. Prescription drug coverage would afford beneficiaries financial protection against the costs associated with all of the major acute care diagnoses. Providing this more comprehensive coverage could save beneficiaries a great deal of money since it would make it less risky for them to have Medicare as their only health insurance. Finally, now would seem to be an opportune time to enact these changes, given the federal budget surplus and the apparent popular goodwill toward ideas aiming to expand Medicare benefits.

The enhanced benefits discussed, however, could be improved by providing a more comprehensive prescription drug benefit. The first useful enhancement would be covering more than 50 percent of prescription costs. A second would be to include prescription drugs in the out-of-pocket cap, so that large prescription drug expenses would be less likely to lead to substantial financial harm. Although both of these modifications would be costly, they would make Medicare coverage more consistent with current employment-based coverage and would better bring it in line with the purpose of insurance.

The second proposal type explored in this paper, premium support, is problematic. It would transform Medicare into a system based much more on competitive markets. Although it is certainly desirable to give beneficiaries an incentive to choose cost-efficient health care plans, many questions remain. First, are beneficiaries sophisticated enough shoppers of health care to choose the plan that is right for them? Second, will plans have enough incentive to provide good quality care when faced with such strong financial incentives to control costs? Third, is it possible to develop effective risk-adjustment formulas so that health plans will not be rewarded for having healthier enrollees? And finally, how can we avoid a situation in which Medicare turns into a two-tier program: one for the well-heeled and another for poorer beneficiaries?

Medicare has made great strides in recent years to become a more efficient program, not only through expanding and improving its managed care offerings but through rationalizing its methods for paying hospitals and physicians. The program is very strong. Enhancing it rather than replacing it with one based on an untested system of premium support would seem to be the next logical step in providing adequate health insurance coverage to Medicare beneficiaries.

NOTES

CHAPTER 3

1. Thomas Rice and Jill Bernstein, "Supplemental Health Insurance for Medicare Beneficiaries," Medicare Brief no. 6, National Academy of Social Insurance, Washington, D.C., November 1999.

2. U.S. General Accounting Office, "Medigap Insurance: Law Has Increased Protection against Substandard and Overpriced Policies," GAO/HRD-87-8, 1986.

3. Although other types of insurance also encourage the use of more services, there is one peculiarity about Medigap: most of the extra costs are borne not by policy owners but by the Medicare program as a whole. Ownership of such policies does indeed result in higher utilization, but since these extra costs mainly are covered by Medicare, the program is essentially subsidizing the purchase of Medigap policies, which would be more expensive (and presumably less appealing) otherwise.

4. Lauren A. McCormack et al., "Medigap Reform Legislation of 1990: Have the Objectives Been Met?" *Health Care Financing Review* 18, no. 1 (Fall 1996): 157–74.

5. Lisa M. Alecxih et al., "Key Issues Affecting Accessibility to Medigap Insurance," Commonwealth Fund, New York, August 1997.

6. Barbara S. Cooper and Margaret H. Davis, "On the Road to Medicare Drug Coverage," paper presented at the Seventh Princeton Conference, sponsored by the Robert Wood Johnson Foundation, Princeton, N.J., May 13, 2000.

7. Rice and Bernstein, "Supplemental Health Insurance for Medicare Beneficiaries."

8. Joanne A. Lamphere et al., "The Surge in Medicare Managed Care: An Update," *Health Affairs* 16, no. 3 (May/June 1997): 127–33.

9. Ibid.

10. Thomas Kornfeld and Marsha Gold, "Is There More or Less Choice?" *Monitoring Medicare+Choice Fast Facts,* no. 1, Mathematica Policy Research, Washington, D.C., December 1999.

11. Ibid.

12. The October 1999 issue of the *Journal of Health Politics, Policy, and Law* (vol. 24, no. 5) was devoted to different views on the managed care backlash.

13. John E. Ware, Jr., et al., "Differences in 4-Year Health Outcomes for Elderly and Poor, Chronically Ill Patients Treated in HMO and Fee-for-Service Systems: Results from the Medical Outcomes Study," *Journal of the American Medical Association* 276 (1996): 1039–47.

14. Robert H. Miller and Harold S. Luft, "Does Managed Care Lead to Better or Worse Quality of Care?" *Health Affairs* 16, no. 5 (September/October 1997): 7–25.

15. See, for example, Kathryn M. Langwell and Jack P. Hadley, "Insights from the Medicare HMO Demonstrations," *Health Affairs* 9, no. 1 (January/February 1990): 74–84.

16. Michael A. Morrisey, Gail A. Jensen, and Stephen E. Henderlite, "Employer-Sponsored Health Insurance for Retired Americans," *Health Affairs* (Spring 1990): 57–73.

17. Rice and Bernstein, "Supplemental Health Insurance for Medicare Beneficiaries."

18. Michael E. Gluck, "A Medicare Prescription Drug Benefit," Medicare Brief no. 1, National Academy of Social Insurance, Washington, D.C., April 1999.

19. Frank McArdle et al., "Retiree Health Coverage: Recent Trends and Employer Perspectives on Future Benefits," Henry J. Kaiser Family Foundation, Menlo Park, Calif., October 1999.

20. Kaiser Family Foundation and Health Research and Educational Trust, *Employer Health Benefits, 1999* (Menlo Park, Calif.: Henry J. Kaiser Family Foundation, 1999).

21. "Retiree Health Insurance: Erosion in Retiree Health Benefits Offered by Large Employers," U.S. General Accounting Office, GAO/T-HEHS-98-110, 1998.

22. Ibid.

23. "Shortchanged: Billions Withheld from Medicare Beneficiaries," Families USA Foundation, Washington, D.C., July 1998.

24. Franklin J. Eppig and George S. Chulis, "Trends in Medicare Supplementary Insurance: 1992–96," *Health Care Financing Review* 19, no. 1 (Fall 1997): 201–6.

25. "Shortchanged: Billions Withheld from Medicare Beneficiaries."

26. Ibid.

27. David J. Gross et al., "Out-of-Pocket Spending by Medicare Beneficiaries Age 65 and Older: Further Analysis of 1997 Projections," paper presented at the Association for Health Services Research Annual Meeting, Washington, D.C., June 1998, prepared by the Public Policy Institute of the American Association of Retired Persons and the Lewin Group, Inc., Washington, D.C., June 23, 1998.

28. U.S. General Accounting Office, "Retiree Health Insurance"; "Health Benefits in 1998" (Washington, D.C.: KPMG Peat Marwick, 1998), n. 22.

29. "Big Increases Set for Medigap Premiums," *Washington Post,* December 21, 1995.

30. R. O. Morgan, "The Medicare-HMO Revolving Door: The Healthy Go In and the Sick Go Out," *New England Journal of Medicine* 337, no. 3 (July 17, 1997): 169–75.

31. Roger Feldman and Bryan Dowd, "Must Adverse Selection Cause Premium Spirals?" *Journal of Health Economics* 10, no. 3 (October 1991): 349–57.

CHAPTER 4

1. Although Part B is voluntary, about 95 percent of beneficiaries choose this benefit because it is so heavily subsidized.

2. For states, the impact of prescription drug copayments would depend on the type of Medicaid coverage. States already pay for prescription drugs for those with full coverage, so Medicare coverage for some of these costs would reduce state outlays. For QMBs, however, who currently do not have coverage for prescription drugs through Medicaid, state costs would rise because states would now be responsible for paying any cost-sharing requirements on drug coverage.

3. This is likely in part because of policy standardization, which makes policy benefits perfectly comparable across companies.

4. Thomas Rice, Marcia L. Graham, and Peter D. Fox, "The Impact of Policy Standardization on the Medigap Market," *Inquiry* 34, no. 2 (Summer 1997): 106–16.

5. George S. Chulis et al., "Health Insurance and the Elderly: Data from MCBS," *Health Care Financing Review* 14, no. 3 (Spring 1993): 163–81; Morrisey, Jensen, and Henderlite, "Employer-Sponsored Health Insurance for Retired Americans."

6. For a comprehensive premium support proposal, see Henry J. Aaron and Robert D. Reischauer, "The Medicare Reform Debate: What Is the Next Step?" *Health Affairs* 14, no. 4 (Winter 1995): 8–30.

7. Marilyn Moon, "Restructuring Medicare: Impacts on Beneficiaries," Urban Institute, Washington, D.C., January 1999.

8. This is not a certainty, however; it is possible that the savings that an employer would receive by enrolling retirees in a managed care plan would exceed the costs associated with losing the subsidy.

9. Aaron and Reischauer, "Medicare Reform Debate"; Marilyn Moon and Karen Davis, "Preserving and Strengthening Medicare," *Health Affairs* 14, no. 4 (Winter 1995): 31–46.

INDEX

Access to health care: Clinton reform proposal and, 166; disparities in, 27–28

Accountability: causes of trend toward, 79–80; effects of, 86; methods of, 81–85; professional vs. market, 79, 121n7

Acute care, vs. prescription drug coverage, 54–55

Administration of Medicare, 101–4; Breaux-Frist proposal and, 125n7, 158–60, 165, 172–73, 181; Clinton reform proposal and, 165; improvement of, approaches to, 104, 125n1; inadequate resources of, 18, 101–3; *See also* Health Care Financing Administration (HCFA)

Administrative costs of Medicare, 40f; premium support proposal and, 172–73; vs. private insurance, 18; trends in, 102f

Adverse selection, problem of, 26, 107n9; Medicare features guarding against, 27; premium support proposals and, 68; prescription drug coverage and, 53; private health plans and, 32, 109n24; risk adjustment and,

32–33; supplemental insurance and, 27; voluntary drug benefit and, 59

African Americans: civil rights of, Medicare and, 76; health services for, compared to whites, 64, 65f; health status of, compared to whites, 65, 118n11

Age. *See* Eligibility age; Retirement age

Agency for Health Care Policy and Research, 85

Alliance of Community Health Plans, 123n36

Antifraud measures, 103

"Attained-age" rating, 197

Balanced Budget Act of 1997 (BBA), 3–4; and beneficiary education, 96; and cost-containment provisions, 8, 131; and geographic disparities, reduction in, 148–49; and Medicare + Choice program, 11, 13, 92, 97–98, 147; and Medicare managed care plans, 199; and National Bipartisan Commission, 135; and Part B financing, 39, 110n3; and payments to plans, 147–48; and

Note: Page numbers followed by letters *f, n,* and *t* refer to figures, notes, and tables, respectively.

ABOUT THE BACKGROUND
PAPER AUTHORS

LISA POTETZ is director of public policy research at the March of Dimes. She prepared this paper as an independent health policy analyst. She has served on the majority staff of the House Ways and Means Committee (1993–95) and the Senate Finance Committee (1989–93), focusing on Medicare policy and health care reform issues, and has worked as senior associate director for policy at the American Hospital Association, senior analyst at the Prospective Payment Assessment Commission, and analyst at the Congressional Budget Office.

THOMAS RICE is professor and chair of the Department of Health Services at the UCLA School of Public Health. Previously, he served on the faculty at the University of North Carolina School of Public Health. In 1988, he received the Association for Health Services Research Young Investigator Award, given to the outstanding health services researcher in the United States age thirty-five or under, and in 1992, he received the Thompson Prize from the Association of University Programs in Health Administration, awarded annually to the outstanding health services researcher in the country age forty or under. He is the author of *The Economics of Health Reconsidered* (Health Administration Press, 1998).